The Meat Effect

The Meat Effect

What Eating Animals Does Inside the Human Body

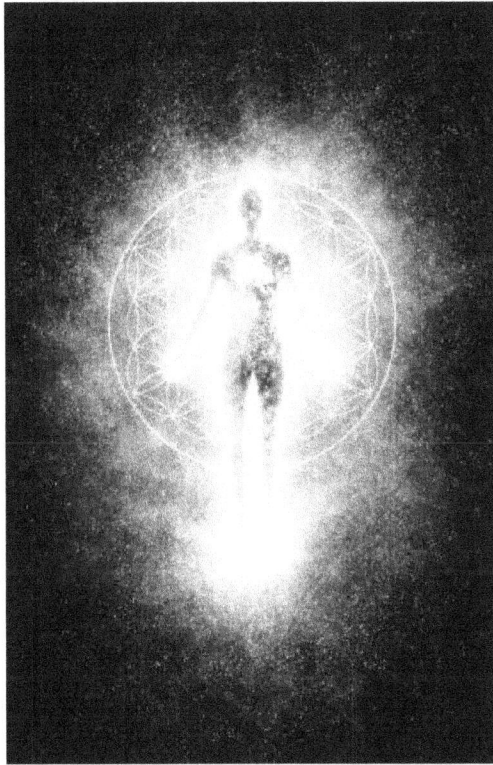

The Biological Evidence Linking Animal Foods to Chronic Illness

**By Jesse J. Jacoby &
Anthony Lowther**

The Meat Effect

Soulspire Publishing
Truckee, CA, 96161

ISBN: 978-1-968660-34-5
Library of Congress Control Number: 2012921011
Dewey CIP: 641.563   **OCLC:** 213839254

Cover art, font, and layout are all original art by: Abdul Rehman

Wholesalers to book trade: Nelson's Books and Ingram
Available through Amazon.com, BarnesAndNoble.com

Dedication

To the Light within all life, and pulse that moves through every creature, leaf, and breath of air.

May this work serve as a reminder that we are not separate from nature but made of the same living current that feeds the stars.

To all children, whose laughter keeps our hearts honest and awake. May you inherit a world cleaner, kinder, and more radiant than the one we were given.

To every seeker walking the path of purification. This book is for you.

May this information remind you that healing is not found in complexity, but in the simple return to truth.

Acknowledgments

This book was born through years of lived experiment, observation, and devotion.

To the clients and friends who trusted us with their healing journeys, your transformations gave these pages their meaning.

To the teachers and pioneers whose works lit the way, Hilton Hotema, Arnold Ehret, Aris Latham, and the many unnamed healers who remembered before us that the human body is a microcosm of the cosmos.

To our community of readers, whose curiosity and courage continue to expand this movement of conscious nourishment. Thank you for proving that awareness can transform culture.

Finally, to the Source of all inspiration, the quiet intelligence that writes through us when we are still enough to listen. May this work serve that current well.

Table of Contents

Introduction: The Flesh of the Matter

For centuries, we have been told that meat makes us strong. That a slab of flesh on the plate is a symbol of vitality, masculinity, survival, and success. Generations have passed down this belief like scripture that protein equals power and meat equals health. The story is so deeply woven into culture that questioning the narrative feels almost heretical. Yet, behind this story lies a quieter, measurable, biochemical reality unfolding within every cell of the body.

When we eat meat, we are not simply consuming protein. We are engaging in a complex chain reaction of chemistry, microbiology, and inflammation that shapes our health from the inside out. Each bite sets off an invisible storm: bacterial endotoxins flooding the bloodstream, ammonia and uric acid taxing the kidneys, acid-forming microbes multiplying in the gut, and oxidized fats disrupting cellular membranes. The body fights back, always striving for balance, but with every meal of animal flesh, that balance becomes harder to maintain.

Inside the colon, where plant fibers once nourished beneficial bacteria, meat leaves emptiness. Without that fiber, putrefaction begins. Proteins rot instead of ferment. Out of that decay arise compounds with names that sound like warnings. These include skatole, indole, and cadaverine, the very chemicals responsible for the smell of death. These toxins are absorbed into the bloodstream, circulate to the liver, and force the body to detoxify what never should have entered in the first place. The result is a subtle, chronic poisoning of our internal environment. One that modern science is finally beginning to measure.

At the microscopic level, the human body does not recognize meat as friend or fuel. Several molecules, including Neu5Gc, TMAO, butyrobetaine, and oxidized cholesterol, act like foreign invaders, igniting immune responses and eroding the delicate lining of arteries. The endothelial cells that once flowed with youthful ease begin to stiffen, the blood grows thicker, and the energy of life slows. Our organs work harder, our microbiome loses harmony, and the silent embers of disease begin to glow.

Yet this is not a book of blame or guilt. This is a book of *understanding* and connecting biology with awareness, and science with compassion. The human body is miraculous in our resilience. Our body wants to heal and purify. When we stop feeding on decay, our bodily systems return to design, clearing the blood, regenerating the gut, and restoring clarity to the mind. The same intelligence that once tried to protect us from the burden of meat will rebuild us the moment we return to life-based nourishment.

This book is not about restriction but is about reconnection. To eat in alignment with vitality is not to give something up but to remember what the body has always known *that life feeds on life, not on death.* The plants, fruits, seeds, and sunlight we are meant to thrive on still wait patiently for our return.

The truth is not hidden in moral arguments or marketing campaigns but is written in biochemistry. When we understand *The Meat Effect*, we understand why the human body thrives when freed from flesh. We learn that energy, clarity, and joy are not found through domination over life, but through harmony with what is living.

In this harmony, the radiant, living intelligence of the plant kingdoms and queendoms, we rediscover the meaning of nourishment.

Part I: Inside the Body – The Biology of Decay

What Happens When Flesh Meets the Human Design

The body is a cathedral of intelligence. A symphony of cells, fluids, and unseen forces working together in exquisite precision. Every thought, heartbeat, and breath depends on this silent harmony. When we eat, we are not simply fueling; we enter communion with life. Each meal is a conversation between matter and spirit. A dialogue that determines whether our systems move toward vitality or toward decay.

For much of human history, we have mistaken the feeling of fullness for the presence of nourishment. We have equated heaviness with strength, mistaking the sedative drag of digestion for satisfaction. Yet beneath the surface, a different story unfolds, one written in molecules, microbes, and energy fields. This is a story that begins not in the mouth, but in the gut, where everything we eat is either converted into living light or buried as metabolic waste.

When meat enters the body, the conversation changes tone. What was once a symphony is now a slow, distorted hum. The digestive tract, designed for fiber and light-filled foods, must now struggle to dismantle dense animal tissue. Hydrochloric acid surges, enzymes scramble to keep up, and the microbiome, our inner ecosystem, shifts toward bacteria that thrive on putrefaction. As flesh is broken down, compounds with ominous names are released. These include skatole, indole, and cadaverine. The chemistry of rot.

These toxins are absorbed into the bloodstream, circulate through the liver, and awaken an ancient defense response we know as inflammation. The immune system, sensing invaders, begins a war that cannot be won. The blood grows cloudy with endotoxins, arteries tighten, mitochondria slow, and life force dims, one meal at a time.

13

This story, however, is not one of hopelessness but of awareness, and of finally seeing what has been hidden in plain sight. Science now confirms what intuition has whispered for generations: *that flesh foods carry a burden the human body was never meant to bear.* From the molecular residue of decay to the inflammatory cascade that follows, each bite of meat leaves a trace, an echo, and a cost.

In the chapters that follow, we will step inside the body, cell by cell, and organ by organ, to witness what truly happens when we consume animal flesh. You will meet the compounds your body must neutralize, the microbes that awaken in your colon, and the biochemical storms that silently shape your energy, mood, and lifespan.

This is a journey of biology. One that reveals how, when we feed on death, the body mirrors what is consumed. When we return to life-based foods, however, plants that pulse with photons, enzymes, and uncorrupted intelligence, the inner cathedral begins to sing again. The light returns. The systems remember. Then the body, once burdened by the weight of flesh, begins to rise again into resonance.

Chapter 1: Anatomy of Truth – Why the Human Body Is Not Designed for Flesh

For centuries, human beings have assumed that our bodies are omnivorous by design. That we are capable, adaptable eaters made to thrive equally on plants and animals. Biology, though, is not determined by culture, and physiology does not bend to habit. The body tells the truth in ways our traditions do not. Every system of human anatomy, from our teeth to our gut, and from our enzymes to our vision, reflects a different story. Not the story of a predator, or an omnivore, but the story of a frugivore. This chapter is a return to that truth. The truth the body never stopped speaking.

Long before industry propaganda, nutritional confusion, and cultural conditioning, the human organism revealed an original blueprint. This is written in our digestive tract, our metabolic chemistry, our salivary enzymes, our endocrine rhythms, and the ecology of the microbiome. Every measurable feature points to the same conclusion: the human being is designed for fruit, leafy greens, roots, nuts, seeds, and tender vegetables, not flesh.

The argument is anatomical, not philosophical. Not ideological but biological. Not emotional but structural. We were never built to eat meat. When we do, the body pays at every level, whether cellular, microbial, neurological, cardiovascular, hormonal, or emotional. This chapter reveals why, and how the evidence has always been in our tissues, awaiting rediscovery.

The Anatomical Map: A Body Built for Plants

No single anatomical feature determines diet, but when every feature points in the same direction, the design becomes unmistakable. Comparative anatomy used for over a century to classify species shows that humans match frugivores and herbivores on every major point.

Below is the anatomical evidence:

1. Teeth, Jaw, and Chewing Physiology

Carnivores possess:

- Sharp fangs.
- Scissor-like bite.
- Jaw motion limited to up-and-down.
- No capacity for lateral grinding.

Omnivores possess:

- Shorter digestive tracts.
- Canine teeth capable of puncture.
- Mixed dentition for omnivorous diets.

Humans possess:

- Small, blunt canines incapable of puncture.
- Flat molars designed for grinding.
- Jaws that move laterally, side-to-side, like Herbivores.
- Chewing patterns optimized for fruit mastication.

We also produce salivary amylase, a carbohydrate-digesting enzyme. Carnivores produce none. Flesh-eaters tear and swallow. Humans chew and grind. The body's intention is clear.

2. Digestive Tract Length and Transit Time

Carnivores have short gastrointestinal tracts, three to six times their body length, to expel rotting protein before bacterial decomposition creates toxicity.

Humans have long digestive tracts that are ten to twelve times our body length, identical to herbivores and frugivores.

When meat enters a long tract, the remnants:

- Putrefies.
- Generates ammonia, cadaverine, and skatole.
- Releases endotoxins.
- Stagnates.
- Acidifies the gut environment.
- Feeds pathogenic bacteria.

No anatomical adaptation counters this. We house decomposition inside us when we consume flesh.

3. Stomach Acidity and Pathogen Defense

Carnivore stomach acid: pH 1

- Designed to dissolve bone and sterilize bacteria.

Human stomach acid: pH 4–5

- Not strong enough to sterilize flesh or kill the pathogens commonly present in raw or cooked meat.

This is why:

- Meat eaters suffer frequent foodborne illness.
- Humans require cooking as a survival mechanism.
- Pathogens survive transit into the intestines.

We rely on external tools such as fire, knives, and heat to compensate for what we lack internally. No predator needs such assistance.

4. Sweating and Cooling Mechanisms

Carnivores pant through the tongue. Herbivores and frugivores sweat through millions of pores.

Humans:
- Sweat through 2–4 million eccrine glands.
- Cool like a distance-frugivore.
- Lack the evaporative panting mechanism of carnivores.

This is the physiology of heat dispersion for long foraging, not hunting and killing prey.

5. Vision: The Language of Color

Carnivores see primarily motion and contrast. Humans see full-spectrum color, identical to fruit-eating primates.

We were designed to detect:
- Ripeness.
- Freshness.
- Subtle gradients of plant pigmentation.
- Biophotonic glow.
- Vibrational quality of living matter.

Meat offers none of these cues. Fruit offers all.

6. Instinctive Appetite

Give a toddler:
- An apple.
- A live rabbit.

The child will eat the apple and pet the rabbit. No matter the culture. No matter the upbringing. Instinct betrays biology: Humans do not see prey, we see life.

7. Microbiome Composition

Frugivores host large populations of:

- Bifidobacteria.
- Lactobacillus.
- Prevotella.
- Butyrate-producers.

Humans share this exact profile.

Carnivores host:

- Fusobacterium.
- Clostridium perfringens.
- Bilophila wadsworthia.
- Sulfur-reducing bacteria.

These microbes overgrow in humans only when we eat meat, creating inflammation, leaky gut, and endotoxemia. Our microbiome reveals our design. We are microbially aligned with the fruit-eater lineage, not the predator lineage.

The Physiology of Misalignment

The moment meat enters a human digestive system; our biology must compensate for the mismatch. This compensation is what the meat-eating world mistakenly describes as *"normal digestion,"* but this is not normal.

Below are the physiological consequences built into the design:

1. Putrefaction Begins Within Hours

The long human digestive tract allows flesh to:

- Rot.
- Ferment.
- Release sulfurous gases.
- Generate carcinogenic amines.

These compounds are identical to those produced in decomposing corpses.

2. Endotoxins Enter the Bloodstream

Meat, even cooked, introduces lipopolysaccharides (LPS), triggering:

- Inflammation.
- Immune activation.
- Oxidative stress.
- Mitochondrial slowdown.
- Vascular injury.

This is measurable within two to six hours of eating meat.

3. TMAO Formation

Carnitine and choline from animal tissue convert to trimethylamine oxide (TMAO), causing:

- Endothelial dysfunction
- Heightened clot risk
- Atherosclerosis.

Plant versions of these nutrients do not generate TMAO.

4. Chronic Acid Load

Meat metabolism produces:

- Uric acid.
- Sulfuric acid.
- Phosphoric acid.
- Nitric acid.

These acids:

- Pull minerals from bone.
- Deplete electrolytes.
- Acidify the lymph.
- Burden the kidneys.

This is why heavy meat eaters often feel:

- Thirsty.
- Depleted.
- Cramp-prone.
- Fatigued.
- Inflamed.

The body is using our own tissues to buffer dietary acid.

5. Neurological Impact

Byproducts of meat digestion enter blood & reach the brain:

- Ammonia.
- Endotoxins.
- Inflammatory cytokines.
- Iron-induced oxidative stress.

This creates:

- Anxiety.
- Irritability.
- Brain fog.
- Neuroinflammation.
- Sleep disruption.

Meat clouds the electrical field of the brain.

The Biochemical Illusion of Strength

For those who claim, *"I feel stronger eating meat,"* science reveals the real mechanism:

- Cortisol spikes.
- Adrenaline surges.
- Dopamine rises.
- The sympathetic nervous system activates.
- Pathogenic gut microbes are fed.

This is stimulation, not nourishment. This is addiction, not vitality. This is the fight-or-flight chemistry masquerading as strength.

When they stop eating meat:

- Detox begins.
- Pathogens starve.
- Withdrawal sets in.
- The adrenals recalibrate.

This discomfort is misinterpreted as "needing meat," yet they never needed meat. They required microbial balance, electrolytes, healing, and time.

The Ancient Arguments Are Not Science

The meat narrative rests on flawed myths:

- "Cavemen ate meat."
- "We evolved big brains from flesh."
- "Meat is bioavailable nutrition."
- "Meat gives complete protein."
- "We need heme iron."
- "There is no B12 in plants."

Every one of these claims is disproven by modern research on:

- Hominin dentition.
- Isotope analysis.
- Microbiome evolution.
- Nutrient metabolism.
- Mitochondrial biology.
- Endocrinology.

We did not grow large brains from flesh. We grew them from glucose, starch, fruit, algae-derived DHA, oxygen, and light.

The anthropological truth is far clearer:

- Early humans ate meat occasionally, out of scarcity, not design.

- Longevity did not rise until animal consumption fell.

Eat Alike for All Blood Types

We feel called to bring awareness to the fact that all of us have the same anatomical and physiological make-up, and our blood type does not in any way change how our body absorbs, digests, excretes, or is nourished. Elephants possess serologic evidence of different blood groups. All primates have presence of ABO polymorphism. There are eleven major blood group systems in cattle.

Every species has a variety of blood types, yet humans are the only ones impressionable enough to be fooled into believing they should be eating different food groups because of diverse antigens in their blood.

All cows naturally eat grass. Elephants and primates tend to eat the same, no matter what their blood type. Why would a human be encouraged to eat out of alignment with their anatomy for an idea that is not backed or supported by common sense simply because someone thought of this?

What is most important for every one of us is that we eat in a way that best supports human anatomy, biology, and physiology. This can be deciphered as eating in a way that does the least amount of damage to our blood, cells, and tissues, and requires minimal energy for digestion.

The Conclusion of Anatomy

Every design feature speaks the same message:

- Humans are frugivores by birth.
- Humans are herbivores by physiology.
- Humans are not meat-eaters by nature.

Every deviation from that design carries a cost. The cost is inflammation, stagnation, endotoxemia, acidity, vascular damage, and accelerated aging.

Before toxins enter the bloodstream, the body whispers the truth in craving patterns, digestive distress, and mood shifts. Before chronic disease forms, the microbiome reveals the early imbalance. Before diagnosis, the light dims from the blood.

The body is always telling us what we were made for. We require fruit, greens, living water, nuts, roots, seeds, and sunlight. We are designed for life. We were never designed for flesh.

Chapter 2: What Happens When Meat Hits the Body

The Science of Digestion, Decay, & the Unchanging Laws of Biology

Whether raised on a green hillside or confined to an industrial feedlot, every animal body, once consumed, becomes subject to the same biochemical laws. The moment meat enters the human digestive tract; this is no longer a story of origin but a story of *chemistry*. No amount of grass-fed purity, organic labeling, or humane certification can change what happens next. The molecular composition of flesh, including dense proteins, animal fats, cholesterol, and microbial remnants, activates a cascade of physiological events that the human body must work tirelessly to manage.

The First Stage: Digestion Under Duress

The mouth prepares the meal with minimal salivary enzymes; unlike herbivores, humans produce very little amylase or protease here. As the meat descends into the stomach, hydrochloric acid is secreted in heavy concentration, forcing the stomach to reach near the lowest possible pH threshold. This acid bath attempts to denature tough animal proteins such as collagen, elastin, and myoglobin, unraveling them into amino acid chains. This process demands enormous energy and time. Digestion of flesh can occupy the stomach for four to six hours before even reaching the small intestine.

During this time, putrefaction begins. Even before the body fully extracts nutrients, anaerobic bacteria start fermenting the proteins, releasing ammonia, hydrogen sulfide, and methyl mercaptan. These are gases associated with decay. What feels like fullness is, in truth, the body straining under biochemical load.

The Second Stage: The Burden of Breakdown

Once the partially digested mass, called *chyme*, enters the small intestine, pancreatic enzymes try to finish the job. The proteins are cleaved into smaller fragments, and fats are emulsified by bile. Animal tissue contains no fiber. This means there is nothing to sweep or stimulate peristalsis, so the movement slows. Transit time increases, and what should be a clean exchange becomes a prolonged stagnation.

As the residues linger, they ferment and rot. The microbes feeding on this matter produce compounds such as skatole, indole, and cadaverine. These are literally the same chemicals that emanate from decomposing flesh. These molecules are absorbed through the intestinal wall, traveling to the liver, where they must be neutralized and excreted. The detoxification process consumes glutathione and other antioxidants, depleting the body's natural defense systems.

This sequence unfolds identically regardless of whether the meat came from a factory-farmed cow or a grass-fed one. The bacterial breakdown of animal protein and fat always yields ammonia, putrefactive amines, and sulfurous toxins. The chemistry is not discriminatory. This digestive outcome is dictated by structure, not source.

The Endotoxin Effect

Alongside these byproducts, the cell walls of bacteria that inhabit or contaminate meat (even after cooking) release lipopolysaccharides known as endotoxins. These molecules enter the bloodstream through the intestinal wall, especially when that lining is compromised by inflammation. Once in circulation, endotoxins trigger a full-body immune response, leading to fatigue, fever, and the chronic low-grade inflammation now linked to heart disease, diabetes, and cognitive decline.

Cooking meat does not neutralize these toxins; in fact, the heating process often ruptures bacterial membranes, *releasing* more endotoxin material into the food. Even the most meticulously prepared steak carries a microscopic residue of these inflammatory triggers.

Acid, Ammonia, and the Exhausted Blood

The digestion of animal protein produces acidic byproducts such as uric acid, phosphoric acid, and sulfuric acid, all of which must be neutralized by drawing alkaline minerals from bones and tissues. This is one reason why high-meat diets correlate with calcium loss and kidney strain. Uric acid is the same substance that crystallizes in joints as gout. Ammonia, another breakdown product, is neurotoxic and places stress on the liver's urea cycle.

Inside the blood, these compounds act like static, disrupting the smooth communication between cells. Mitochondria, the energy generators, slow their output in the presence of oxidative stress. The overall electrical potential of the body, our true vitality, declines.

This happens in every human body, every time meat is consumed. Grass-fed, free-range, or organic makes no biological difference. The source of the tissue cannot change the fundamental composition or the reactions being provoked within us.

The Great Illusion of "Healthy Meat"

Marketing has done what chemistry cannot: *rebranded flesh as a nutrient*. Words like *pasture-raised*, *ethically sourced*, and *clean protein* attempt to distance consumers from the reality that meat, no matter of origin, decomposes in the same way inside the gut.

A cow's diet of grass does not remove uric acid, cholesterol, or the bacterial remnants that cling to tissues. Once cooked and ingested, these compounds ignite the same internal chemistry of inflammation. What differs is only the external story. The narrative that makes people feel better about eating what their biology cannot truly handle.

The Unchanging Law of Matter

The human body operates by immutable principles. Flesh is dense, anaerobic matter that demands decomposition before assimilation. Plants, by contrast, come pre-structured for symbiosis and are filled with enzymes, water, fiber, and light-coded nutrients. One leads to fermentation and decay, the other to vitality and flow.

This is not a moral argument, but a biochemical one. Nature does not judge but does measure. Every cell, molecule, and organ system keeps score of what enters. The equations of digestion do not bend for belief or branding.

When we eat meat, the body must convert death into life. While attempting heroically to accomplish this, every attempt leaves a trace in the blood, tissues, and energy that animates our being.

In the chapters ahead, we will explore what those traces mean: the hidden endotoxins in the bloodstream, acid load on the kidneys, damage to the endothelial lining, and slow dimming of vitality that follows. Understanding *The Meat Effect* is not about blame but is about reclaiming truth from illusion and giving the body the freedom to remember what real nourishment feels like.

Chapter 3: The Toxic Harvest

Endotoxins, Bowel Byproducts, & the Blood Beneath the Flesh

Digestion begins in the stomach. What happens next, within the intestines, bloodstream, and lymphatic channels, determines whether food becomes life or burden. When the meal contains animal flesh, the transformation leans toward burden. The chemistry of decomposition continues long after swallowing, and the invisible microbes that inhabit the gut become architects of disease.

The Microbes of Decay

In a body nourished by plants, the gut is a garden. Microbes feast on fiber, producing short-chain fatty acids like butyrate that heal the colon and regulate immunity. In a body fed on flesh, however, that garden turns into a graveyard. Fiber disappears, oxygen levels drop, and anaerobic bacteria rise from the depths. These are species that thrive on putrefaction rather than life.

These bacteria, such as *Clostridium, Bacteroides, Fusobacterium,* and others, feed on the proteins, fats, and secondary metabolites of animal tissue. In breaking them down, they excrete amines, phenols, ammonia, and hydrogen sulfide, substances toxic to human cells. What these microbes release does not remain in the gut. Their waste seeps through the intestinal wall, hitching a ride into the bloodstream to mingle with our own chemistry.

The body then faces a double burden: the toxins from the food and microbial waste created while digesting. These microbial metabolites, being skatole, indole, putrescine, cadaverine, and phenylacetate are lipophilic, meaning they dissolve in fat and easily cross into tissues and organs. Once in circulation, they irritate the liver, kidneys, and brain, forcing the body to detoxify the microbial sewage.

Endotoxemia: When Microbial Waste Enters the Blood

The intestinal lining is meant to be a sacred boundary, separating the outside world from our inner sanctum. When inflamed by acid-forming diets and meat-based residues, however, that lining becomes porous. This nurtures a condition now known as *leaky gut syndrome*. Through these microscopic gaps slip lipopolysaccharides (LPS), fragments of bacterial cell walls also known as endotoxins.

Even tiny amounts of endotoxin in the blood can trigger a systemic immune reaction. The body interprets this as infection. White blood cells surge, inflammatory cytokines rise, and the liver works overtime to neutralize the assault. The person may never feel acutely ill, but fatigue, brain fog, joint pain, and chronic inflammation quietly take root.

Studies have shown that after consuming a high-fat or meat-based meal, levels of endotoxin in the bloodstream rise significantly within hours. This is not infection from the outside but contamination from within.

Chyle: The Milky Mirror of Digestion

After a meal, fats and fat-soluble compounds are absorbed into the lymphatic system in the form of a milky substance called chyle. This is the intermediary between what we eat and what becomes our blood. In a healthy body, nourished by fruits, vegetables, and whole plant foods, chyle is light, clean, and filled with living enzymes. We observe a luminescent fluid carrying the potential of vitality.

When a meal contains meat, dairy, or cooked animal fat, the chyle thickens, color darkens, odor turns sour, and breakdown accelerates. The lipids carried are oxidized, cholesterol is destabilized, and collected bacterial endotoxins begin to ferment within.

As chyle travels through the lymphatic channels toward the bloodstream, instead of pristine nutrients, degraded matter is delivered. Ancient healers once said that the purity of one's blood could be read in the clarity of the chyle. They were not wrong.

Modern microscopy reveals that those who consume high amounts of animal products have cloudier, more viscous lymphatic fluid. Their chyle decomposes faster, forming what early naturopathic physicians called "lymphatic sludge". A slow-moving, congested current of waste. This sluggish flow diminishes oxygen transport and immune efficiency, leaving the body heavy, tired, and toxic.

Blood as Biography

Once the chyle merges with the bloodstream, this becomes the medium of life. We can perceive this as the river that feeds every cell. The composition of that river reflects the quality of what enters. In those who consume plants, the blood remains lighter and more alkaline, with plasma rich in antioxidants, structured water, and nutrient ions. In those who consume meat, the blood grows thicker, more acidic, and filled with residues of uric acid, ammonia, and lipid peroxides.

Microscopic analysis reveals a telling difference: meat eaters show red blood cells that clump and lose their electrical charge, a condition called *rouleaux formation*. This stacking limits oxygen transport and increases the risk of clotting, fatigue, and circulatory distress. In contrast, plant-based eaters display free-floating, vibrant cells with strong zeta potential. This is an indicator of high electrical vitality.

The chemistry of blood mirrors the chemistry of diet. Flesh leads to coagulation, stagnation, and decay; plants lead to flow, charge, and life.

The Quiet Consequence

The tragedy of the modern diet is that most people never see what happens inside them. They feel the temporary fullness and mistake this for nourishment. They may not feel sick, yet their blood tells another story of the slow corrosion of vitality beneath the surface.

The microbes feeding on decay do not rest; they produce continuous waste. The liver and kidneys filter relentlessly, but the cost is cumulative. Each meat-based meal adds another layer of burden. More ammonia to neutralize, more acids to buffer, and more microbial toxins to capture before they reach the brain.

This is the unseen cost of eating flesh: the transformation of the gut from garden to graveyard, of the lymph from living milk to decaying residue, and of the blood from current to coagulation.

Toward a Cleaner Flow

The good news is that the body never forgets how to heal. When the source of burden is removed, the microbial ecosystem rebalances. Fiber returns, fermentation shifts from putrid to probiotic, and the chyle regains clarity. Within weeks of abstaining from animal foods, the blood begins to clear. pH rises, inflammatory markers drop, and the light returns to the plasma. Life always moves toward purification when given the chance.

The next step in this journey is to understand the forces that keep that burden alive. These are the acids, endotoxins, and the false sense of strength that meat delivers while quietly robbing vitality. In the chapters ahead, we will explore how this internal toxicity spreads to the body's major systems, the heart, brain, and gut, and how to reverse the damage through the living intelligence of plants.

Chapter 4: The Acid Load

*How Flesh Foods Steal Minerals, Feed Acidic Microbes, and
Dehydrate the Human Terrain*

The body is designed to live in balance. I am not writing solely about emotional or energetic balance, but chemical balance. Every enzyme, cell, and electrical pulse within us depends on a narrow range of pH and mineral equilibrium. When this harmony shifts toward acidity, life force begins to drain away like current through a frayed wire. Among all the dietary forces that pull us toward that acidic edge, none is stronger than meat.

Acid by Design

Animal flesh is inherently acid-forming. The proteins contain large quantities of the sulfur-bearing amino acids, methionine and cysteine, which, when metabolized, produce sulfuric acid. The nucleic acids degrade into uric acid, phospholipids into phosphoric acid, and nitrogen content into ammonia. Each of these compounds must be buffered, neutralized, or excreted to protect the body from acidosis.

To do this, the body borrows from our own mineral reserves. Calcium, magnesium, potassium, and sodium, the very electrolytes that keep our hearts beating and nerves firing, are pulled from bones, muscles, and blood plasma to restore chemical neutrality. The result is a subtle but chronic mineral depletion.

What is often called "fatigue," "low energy," or "craving salt" is often the cry of a system trying to maintain electrical stability amid an acid storm.

The Arrival of Acid-Forming Bacteria

When meat enters the digestive tract, this not only acidifies the environment chemically but also transforms the biology. The microbes that thrive in this terrain are not the friendly, fiber-loving species that create butyrate and harmony; they are acidogenic bacteria, organisms that flourish in low-oxygen, low-fiber conditions.

Species such as *Clostridium*, *Bacteroides*, and certain *Lactobacillus* strains begin to dominate. They ferment amino acids and fatty residues, producing lactic acid, formic acid, and butyric derivatives that further acidify the gut lumen. The once-neutral terrain becomes a breeding ground for acid-forming colonies whose waste creates irritation, leaky membranes, and inflammation.

This microbial shift is not just about digestion but changes the internal ecosystem of the entire body. Blood pH is tightly regulated, but the interstitial fluids, where our cells live, become progressively acidic. The electrical exchange between cells slows; enzymes misfire; and detoxification stalls.

While cooking meat alters the surface microbiota, the problem is amplified when meat is consumed raw. This is a growing trend among those following carnivore or *"ancestral"* diets. Raw flesh carries live bacterial species from the animal's own gut and skin, including acid-forming strains and opportunistic pathogens. Once introduced to the human terrain, these microbes adapt, proliferate, and feed on nitrogenous waste. Their metabolic byproducts such as organic acids, hydrogen sulfide, and amines, degrade the mucosal lining and further consume the very minerals needed to restore balance.

Why the Modern Carnivore Craves Electrolytes

If we step back, the irony becomes almost poetic. We see the same influencers who advocate for high-meat diets are now also promoting endless electrolyte powders, salt solutions, and mineral blends. They claim that the modern person is *"under-salted"*, yet their own biochemistry is what drives the depletion.

These are some of the reasons why:

• The acid-forming bacteria that thrive on a meat-based diet consume and neutralize electrolytes, using sodium, potassium, and magnesium as buffers against their own waste.

• The acidic residues from protein metabolism force the body to leach these minerals from tissues to maintain blood pH around 7.4.

• As calcium is withdrawn from bone, and magnesium from muscles, the blood temporarily stabilizes at the expense of long-term structure and hydration.

This is why those following heavy flesh-based regimens often experience muscle cramps, palpitations, dizziness, and dry skin. Their bodies are fighting an invisible battle for balance, one that no amount of supplemental salts can truly fix. They are pouring water into a bucket full of holes.

Electrolyte powders become a bandage for the very wound the diet is creating. The cycle perpetuates: meat → acid → mineral loss → supplementation → continued depletion.

The Desert Within

Water follows minerals. When electrolytes are lost, the body's ability to hold structured water declines. This is the crystalline matrix that gives tissues vitality. Hydration is not about how much water we drink, but how well our cells can *retain*. Acid-forming diets dissolve that structure, turning the inner ocean into a stagnant swamp.

Microscopically, this can be seen in the loss of cell membrane potential. The more acidic the environment, the less charge each cell holds. Communication falters. Electrical impulses slow. The body becomes dehydrated from within, even as people drink endlessly from plastic bottles.

In contrast, plant-based diets restore hydration naturally. The organic potassium, magnesium, and calcium in fruits and greens re-establish the mineral charge that binds water to cells. Fiber holds moisture in the gut, while alkalizing plant compounds encourage the return of beneficial microbes that create a gentle, oxygen-rich environment. This is how the body reclaims our rivers and restores flow.

Acid Is Decay, Not Strength

For decades, the story of strength has been told through the lens of meat: the hunter's meal, the warrior's fuel, and the ancestral diet of the "fit," but acid is not power; this is corrosion. True vitality comes from supporting the body through mineral harmony.

The body does not thrive in an acidic swamp. We thrive in an alkaline spring. The muscles that appear *"hardened"* by a meat-heavy diet often mask internal rigidity: calcified arteries, stiff fascia, and dehydrated cells. The outward image of power hides the inward erosion of balance.

Restoring the Mineral Symphony

When we remove flesh from the plate, the terrain begins to shift almost immediately. The acid-forming bacteria lose their food supply and recede. The body stops consuming our own minerals to neutralize their waste. Within days, urine pH begins to rise, signaling that buffering minerals are being conserved rather than sacrificed.

Green juices, fruits, sea vegetables, and sprouts replenish the electrolyte matrix naturally. The cells rehydrate. The blood regains flow. The electrical field that animates every living process grows brighter, stronger, and more coherent.

We are returning to the body's natural design: a terrain of oxygen, minerals, and light. The body was never meant to run on acid. We are designed to run on current.

From Acid to Alchemy

Every transformation begins with awareness. When we see the body not as a machine but as an ecosystem, we realize that every meal is a message. Acidic inputs invite acidic life forms; alkalinity invites renewal. The bacteria we cultivate reflect the environment we create.

To eat meat is to feed the agents of decay. To eat plants is to nourish the architects of life. One pulls minerals out, the other draws light in. One drains, the other regenerates.

In the end, the chemistry is simple. The body keeps score of everything we eat, and the score is written in charge, flow, and radiance.

Chapter 5: Cholesterol & the Fragile Artery

*The Difference Between the Cholesterol We Create and the
Cholesterol We Consume*

Cholesterol has been both demonized and defended for
decades, yet few people understand the true nature of this
molecule. Within our body, cholesterol is not the villain but
is a vital molecule, a soft golden wax synthesized by our
own cells. This forms the membranes of every living cell,
aids in hormone production, and helps the brain maintain
structure and signaling. In natural, internal form, cholesterol
is an *ally of life*.

When cholesterol enters the body from outside,
however, being sourced from cooked animal tissue, eggs,
and dairy, this becomes a foreign lipid carrying the imprint
of death, oxidation, and inflammation. The difference
between the cholesterol we create and the cholesterol we
consume is the difference between pure spring water and
stagnant runoff: one is living, self-regulated, and essential;
the other introduces chaos to the system.

The Body's Own Cholesterol: An Intelligent Design

Every healthy liver produces all the cholesterol the body
could ever need, generating typically around one to two
grams per day. This process is tightly self-regulated: when
the body has enough, production slows; when more is
needed (for cellular repair, hormone synthesis, or membrane
renewal), the liver increases output.

In a well-balanced, plant-based body, this cholesterol
moves through the bloodstream packaged in high-density
lipoproteins (HDL), serving as a recycling agent and
antioxidant. The membranes of every cell shimmer with just
enough of this natural lipid to maintain flexibility and
electrical stability.

Cholesterol is a living material, continuously produced, used, and reabsorbed in harmony with the body's needs. This is endogenous cholesterol. The kind the body makes for us, from within. This form is clean, responsive, and alive.

The Foreign Invader: Dietary Cholesterol

When we ingest meat, eggs, or dairy, we introduce dietary cholesterol. This is a compound that has already undergone oxidation from exposure to air, light, and heat. Cooking animal fat turns cholesterol into oxysterols and cholesterol aldehydes, molecules foreign to the human body. Once absorbed, these unstable lipids embed into cell membranes, damaging the delicate phospholipid bilayer and reducing membrane fluidity.

The liver was never designed to handle *pre-formed cholesterol*, so we cannot regulate or modify this influx. Instead, the body must store, excrete, or neutralize. Most travels through the bloodstream in low-density lipoproteins (LDL), where this easily becomes oxidized. Once oxidized, these particles no longer deliver nutrients, they become inflammatory agents, triggering the immune system to deploy macrophages that engulf the damaged lipids.

This process leads to foam cell formation, arterial plaque, and the slow erosion of the endothelium. This is the single-cell-thick lining that protects every artery in the body. The arteries stiffen, their flexibility fades, and what was once a flowing river becomes a narrow, hardened channel.

Endothelial Injury: The First Crack in the Current

The endothelium is a masterpiece of design. This is the shimmering film of living intelligence that senses blood flow, pressure, and chemistry. This layer of cells regulates nitric oxide production, controls dilation and constriction, and keeps the blood from clotting unnecessarily. Yet this film is delicate and is easily damaged by oxidized cholesterol, high saturated fats, and post-meal endotoxins.

After a single meal rich in animal fat, studies show a measurable decline in endothelial function within hours. The arteries literally lose their ability to relax. The body's internal current slows and the life force that flows through blood becomes turbulent. Over time, this turbulence fosters micro-injuries where oxidized lipids and calcium deposit and form the earliest stages of atherosclerosis.

The problem is not cholesterol but the quality, source, and state of that cholesterol.

The Chemistry of Decay

In raw or cooked animal tissue, cholesterol is bound to triglycerides and phospholipids that oxidize easily. When exposed to air and heat, they generate peroxides, free radicals, and aldehydes. These reactive molecules damage DNA, proteins, and cell membranes. Once these oxidized fats enter circulation, they interfere with the body's natural lipid signaling.

Unlike plant fats, which carry antioxidants like tocopherols, carotenoids, and polyphenols, animal fats are largely devoid of protective compounds. Thus, the body must supply our own antioxidants, vitamin E, glutathione, and superoxide dismutase, to quench the oxidative stress. Over time, this constant depletion accelerates aging, dulls the skin, and inflames the cardiovascular system.

The Myth of "Good" Cholesterol Foods

The wellness industry has repackaged meat, butter, and eggs as *"nutrient-dense"* sources of cholesterol and fat, arguing that dietary cholesterol has little effect on blood cholesterol. But this misunderstanding arises from short-term studies that fail to measure oxidation, inflammation, or long-term endothelial damage.

When we look deeper, beyond the marketing and numbers, the reality is clear: *dietary cholesterol is not neutral.* This is a foreign lipid that must be transported, managed, and detoxified. The more we consume, the more oxidative waste our bodies must clear. The more energy we spend clearing waste, the less we have for regeneration.

The Light and the Lipid

Plant-based diets, rich in chlorophyll, fiber, and antioxidants, allow the body's own cholesterol production to stabilize naturally. LDL levels drop, HDL levels become more efficient, and endothelial repair accelerates. The arteries regain elasticity, and nitric oxide, the molecule of flow, increases. The blood becomes lighter, heart beats easier, and skin regains luster.

This is not just the absence of disease but is the return of light to the lipid layer. Every cell membrane begins to resonate with clarity again. The internal waters clear. The body stops fighting against our own cells.

Two Forms of Cholesterol, Two Outcomes

Endogenous (self-made) cholesterol:

• Produced by the liver in the exact amounts required for repair, hormone synthesis, and membrane fluidity.

• Production down-regulates when supply is sufficient and up-regulates when the body calls for more.

• In a well-balanced, plant-based physiology, this native cholesterol circulates efficiently, supports cell membranes, and contributes to vascular resilience.

Dietary (foreign) cholesterol:

• Introduced from meat, eggs, and dairy, often already oxidized by air and heat, arriving as unstable lipids that embed in membranes and travel primarily in LDL particles.

• These oxidized fragments provoke inflammation, injure the endothelial lining, and promote foam cell formation and plaque. The liver cannot "unsee" or finely regulate this incoming supply, so the burden shifts to transport, storage, and detoxification.

Core distinction:

• Self-produced cholesterol is dynamic, regulated, and supportive of renewal.

• Dietary cholesterol is static, frequently oxidized, and pro-inflammatory, adding workload to the vascular and hepatic systems without offering an essential function that endogenous synthesis does not already provide.

Practical Takeaway

A whole-food, plant-based pattern allows endogenous cholesterol to do a protective job while minimizing foreign, oxidized cholesterol that damages arteries and accelerates aging. The takeaway is simple: the body makes exactly what is required when nourished by clean, living foods.

Every molecule of cholesterol produced internally is made on demand and deconstructed when no longer needed. Dietary cholesterol, however, arrives uninvited and unmanageable, already damaged, already oxidized, and always inflammatory.

The Artery as Oracle

If we could look within the arteries of those who eat a diet rich in animal products, we would see not strength but struggle. A slow narrowing, loss of rhythm, and quiet stiffening. In contrast, the arteries of those who live on plants remain pliable, humming with nitric oxide and flow.

The artery tells the truth and does not lie for industry or ideology. The internal chemistry is recorded, faithfully and without bias. In a silent language, we are taught: *the life we choose to eat becomes the life we allow to move through us.*

Returning to Flow

The good news is that the damage is reversible. Studies show that within weeks of adopting a whole-food, plant-based diet, endothelial function begins to improve. Plaques stabilize or regress, and nitric oxide levels rise. The body operates naturally and heals when we stop the assault.

When we live in alignment with our design, our inner rivers run clear again. The foreign cholesterol disappears. The self-generated, light-infused cholesterol resumes a graceful dance of repair, becoming a conduit for radiance.

Chapter 6: Cooking the Corpse

The Danger of Heat-Damaged Fat & the Manufactured War on Seed Oils

Fire changed the human story, providing warmth, protection, and the illusion that anything placed above became safe to eat. Yet in that flame, the very chemistry of life is undone. When we expose fats, whether plant or animal, to high heat, we fracture their molecular integrity. The bonds that once carried energy and structure turn unstable, creating compounds the body cannot recognize.

Over time, this breakdown became so normal that most forgot this was happening at all. Only when disease began to rise did science start tracing the smoke back to the source.

The Great Diversion: How the Anti-Seed-Oil Movement Began

In recent years, the internet has erupted with a crusade against *"seed oils."* Voices proclaim that vegetable oils are the enemy, that butter and tallow are somehow safer, and that animal fat is *"ancestral fuel."* Few realize how and why this message was amplified.

The modern anti-seed-oil movement arose not from independent science, but as a strategic diversion and redirection of public fear away from the real culprit: *cooked flesh and animal fat.* As decades of research began linking meat consumption to heart disease, cancer, and premature aging, animal agriculture needed a new scapegoat.

They found one in plant oils. By shifting the blame toward sunflower, canola, and soybean oils, they could re-ignite nostalgia for butter, bacon, and beef tallow under the banner of *"real food."* Yet the truth is more nuanced and far less convenient: both damaged seed oils and heated animal fats disrupt human biology. The distinction lies not in the source, but in the chemistry of oxidation.

When Fat Meets Fire

Every fat, whether pressed from an olive or stripped from a cow, contains carbon bonds that store energy. When heated, especially above 180 °C (356 °F), these bonds break apart, forming reactive fragments known as lipid peroxides and aldehydes. These molecules attach to proteins and DNA, creating advanced lipid oxidation end-products (ALEs). These are the fatty cousins of AGEs (advanced glycation end-products). When ingested, these compounds ignite oxidative stress, inflame the endothelium, and alter mitochondrial function. In the bloodstream, they combine with cholesterol to form oxidized LDL, the precise agent that burrows into arterial walls.

Animal fats, however, carry an added burden. Their fatty acids are mostly saturated, meaning they solidify easily and resist movement. Once heated, they form dense, sticky residues that adhere to vessel walls and cell membranes. The result is a slow hardening, not only of arteries, but of the entire energetic system.

The Paradox of "Real Fat"

Proponents of animal fats often claim they are *"more stable"* than plant oils under heat. While true that saturated fats oxidize slightly slower than polyunsaturated ones, what forms in their place is far more noxious. Cooked animal fat produces heterocyclic amines (HCAs), polycyclic aromatic hydrocarbons (PAHs), and oxidized cholesterol derivatives. These compounds are proven to be carcinogenic, mutagenic, and deeply inflammatory.

To imagine their danger, picture the black crust on a grilled steak or the shimmering grease in a frying pan: that sheen is molecular ruin that contains substances so reactive they can mutate DNA and impair mitochondrial respiration.

If overheated vegetable oil is harmful, then the fat that melted from a corpse is exponentially worse. One originates from the alteration of plant lipids, while the other derives from the combustion of animal tissue.

From Sizzle to Sickness

The smell of cooking meat may trigger nostalgia but is chemically identical to the odor of combustion. The same aldehydes and aromatic hydrocarbons found in smoke rise from frying pans. When inhaled, they enter the lungs and bloodstream. If eaten, they line the gut and arteries.

The digestive system must then neutralize this molecular chaos. The liver mobilizes antioxidants, glutathione, and sulfur compounds to break down the poisons. Over time, these reserves are depleted, leading to systemic oxidative stress. The skin dulls, the blood thickens, and the mitochondria, our inner engines, slow under the weight of constant repair.

Why the Body Suffers More from Cooked Animal Fat

Cooked plant oils, though damaging, at least begin as substances designed by nature for light absorption and photosynthetic exchange. Their degradation products can often be filtered and excreted. Cooked animal fats, by contrast, are the remnants of another creature's cellular structure. Once heated, their cholesterol oxidizes into oxysterols, which integrate into our cell membranes and interfere with electrical signaling. These compounds cannot simply be washed away; they embed into the very tissue that sustains us.

Thus, while both heated plant and animal fats harm us, animal fats produce deeper, more persistent forms of decay. The kind that accumulates silently for years before manifesting as disease.

The Mirage of Balance

Many health advocates now suggest a compromise: *"Use both, just avoid processed oils."* Yet the body does not recognize compromise in chemistry. We respond only to molecular truth. Heated fats, of any kind, generate free radicals, endothelial damage, and a burden of detoxification that the liver must endlessly shoulder.

The path to real nourishment is not found in choosing one poison over another, but in stepping back from the fire altogether. The closer food remains to a natural, unheated state, the more all lipids, enzymes, and photons remain intact. True stability comes not from saturation, but from living structure. The molecular coherence found in raw seeds, nuts, avocados, and whole plants.

Fireless Nourishment

When fats are consumed in their raw, plant-based form, they arrive with their own antioxidants, including vitamin E, carotenoids, and chlorophylls that protect them from oxidation and protect us in turn. These lipids integrate smoothly into cell membranes, maintaining flexibility and charge. They fuel the brain without clogging. They support hormones without corrupting them.

In contrast, cooked animal fat is the very definition of biological entropy: once vibrant tissue rendered into oily residue, stripped of life and loaded with toxic byproducts of combustion.

Fire and the Illusion of Safety

Cooking has been celebrated as civilization's greatest innovation but is also how we learned to disguise death. The sear, the aroma, and the caramelized crust are all sensory illusions born of the Maillard reaction. This is the same process that produces brown haze in polluted cities. We do not experience flavor from life but perfume of degradation.

Each browned surface carries thousands of new chemical species, some mildly stimulating, and others outright mutagenic. The nervous system responds to them like narcotics, with a burst of pleasure followed by systemic fatigue. The warmth we associate with comfort food is, biochemically, the warmth of inflammation.

Shifting the Lens Back to Truth

The anti-seed-oil movement was never about saving human health; this was about saving an industry. The propaganda redirected scrutiny away from flesh and toward fields, away from the pan and toward the press. The real question has never been *"which fat is best?"* but *"how far have we drifted from foods that carry living intelligence?"*

Both refined oils and cooked animal fats are echoes of destruction. They are different branches of the same tree of oxidation. The only difference is that one begins in the plant kingdom and loses vitality through processing, while the other begins in the animal kingdom and loses vitality through death and heat.

When we return to foods that have not been burned, bleached, or broken, and when our lipids come from sunlight and chlorophyll rather than smoke and fire, the body responds instantly. The blood thins, mind clears, and electrical pulse of life grows stronger.

The Body's Quiet Instruction

If the oils extracted from plants can harm us once overheated, imagine what happens when the fats of dead animals are cooked, congealed, and carried through our bloodstream. The body tells the truth in every symptom, whether through fatigue, heaviness, or inflammation. These are not punishments but messages.

In that truth lies our invitation: *to leave behind the mythology of "ancestral fats" and reclaim the intelligence of clean, living nourishment.*

Chapter 7: The Bone Broth Myth

Once upon a time, bone broth was sacred. A humble, ancestral remedy. A slow-simmered symbol of nourishment passed from hearth to healing. In the modern age, however, this has been rebranded, commercialized, and elevated to a cure-all that is hailed for containing collagen, minerals, and a supposed regenerative power.

What if we have misunderstood the very biology we are attempting to restore? What if bone broth is not building your body, but is of detriment and a burden?

What Collagen Really Is and Is Not

Collagen is the most abundant protein in the human body, forming the scaffolding of skin, joints, fascia, and connective tissue. In living form, collagen is a triple-helix protein that is structured, intelligent, and electrically active.

The moment collagen is exposed to prolonged heat, especially in boiling water, the composition is denatured (anything heated above 130°F (54°C)). Simmered for hours, collagen is broken down into gelatin, a random assortment of amino acids. These fragments are not inherently harmful, but they are biologically inert. The original structure, which your body can utilize, is gone. You do not ingest collagen and absorb this material whole.

Your body must:

▪ Break the compounds down.

▪ Reassemble them using your own blueprint.

▪ Depend on key cofactors like vitamin C, silica, copper, and zinc.

Without these cofactors, consuming gelatin is like receiving bricks with no blueprint, no builders, and no mortar.

The truth is: collagen must be created, not consumed, and the manufacturing of this protein varies in molecular structure within each species. Human collagen is different than collagen from cows or pigs.

The Hidden Cost of Cooked Bones

Boiling bones does not just extract gelatin.

This process leaches:

- Oxidized fats.

- Heavy metals stored in the marrow.

- Denatured proteins that may trigger immune confusion.

- Inflammatory compounds from animals in confinement.

Perhaps most disturbing: the bones used in most commercial bone broth products are not coming from sacred family farms or wild elk. They are the waste stream of the meat industry.

These bones are:

- Collected in bulk from slaughterhouses and processing plants.

- Often from animals raised in filth, fed GMO grain, injected with antibiotics and growth hormones.

- Rendered from diseased or discarded carcasses that are deemed unfit for meat sale.

- Boiled in massive vats to extract residual protein for consumer resale.

This is not healing but a representation of industrial runoff repackaged as wellness. Bone broth has become a way to profit from what would otherwise be thrown away. This is most often the byproduct of systemic violence, boiled into illusion.

Collagen You Actually Need

The body is equipped with the right tools to create all the collagen we require. What supports real collagen synthesis? This list is living collagen activation with no pot required.

• Vitamin C from camu camu, amla, citrus, and bell peppers.

• Silica from bamboo, horsetail, and cucumber.

• Zinc and copper from pumpkin seeds, nettle, and spirulina.

• Sulfur-rich foods like arugula, broccoli, & mustard greens.

• Hydration & movement to stimulate fascia & lymph flow.

Why Plants Are More Bioavailable

Plant-based collagen builders do not carry foreign DNA.

They come with:

• Enzymes intact.

• Biophotons from sunlight.

• Phytonutrients that co-regulate gene expression.

• No inflammatory baggage.

Your body does not have to work against these foods. You work with them. They whisper instructions to your cells, not just deliver raw materials. Unlike cooked animal protein, they do not create excess acid, uric load, or lymphatic congestion.

The Bone Broth Marketing Machine

The resurgence of bone broth has been heavily pushed by:

• Paleo influencers.

• Collagen supplement companies.

• Meat-based wellness brands.

Much of the science cited is based on short-term trials, extrapolated animal models, and industry-funded claims. When marketing replaces metabolics, sovereignty is lost.

The Way of Living Structure

You do not build life from the dead or rebuild collagen from broken strands. You regenerate by returning to living sources of structure, hydration, and frequency. What you are really seeking is coherence, not collagen.

Let your bones be rebuilt by:

• Grounding on Earth.

• Drinking structured water.

• Moving in spiral patterns.

• Breathing into fascia.

• Eating the colors of the sun.

Closing Reflection

Bone broth does not have to be a villain. This product simply is not the holy grail that persuasive marketing has declared. True regeneration is electrical and begins in the matrix of minerals, enzymes, light, and motion. You do not become whole by boiling bones; you do this by building life from living sources. Feed radiance with what regenerates. Do not sip the myth and expect magic. Feed your body what you can use. Honor your bodily intelligence.

Part II: Systems Under Siege

How Flesh Foods Disrupt the Body's Natural Intelligence

The body is not a collection of parts. We are a continuum of currents. Rivers of blood, networks of nerves, colonies of microbes, and fields of light all synchronized by one invisible principle: *coherence.* When coherence is lost, disease begins long before diagnosis.

Eating flesh dismantles coherence. The breakdown starts small, as an inflamed cell here, or an irritated vessel there, yet these sparks spread until every system of the body begins to echo the same signal of distress. What was once harmony becomes static.

The acids, endotoxins, and oxidized fats born from flesh do not stay confined to the gut. They travel through the bloodstream, alter hormones, disrupt neurotransmitters, and cloud the mind. The body becomes a battlefield of competing chemistries: one fighting for vitality, the other feeding on decay.

Modern science measures this in lab values such as inflammatory markers, lipid peroxides, and elevated uric acid. Beneath those numbers, though, lives a deeper story: *the dimming of the body's electrical potential.* Every organ becomes less efficient, and every signal less clear. The gut loses our garden, the brain loses our calm, the heart loses rhythm, and the hormones lose their song.

This part of the book is a descent into those systems, not to linger in pathology, but to understand where and how the disruption begins, so that repair can follow. For every system that falls under siege, there exists an equal and opposite intelligence within us capable of restoring order when we cease to feed the enemy and return to foods that align with the body's design.

Here, we will explore:

• How the gut becomes the first battlefield, inflamed, stripped of allies, and overrun by the microbes of decay.

• How the brain, bathed in inflammatory molecules, loses clarity and emotional stability.

• How the heart, starved of nitric oxide and burdened by oxidized cholesterol, stiffens until can no longer expand with joy.

•How the hormonal network, driven by acid and stress, ages prematurely and mistakes stimulation for strength.

The war within us is silent but visible in every modern illness. A resolution lies not in medicine but in the remembrance of what life feeds life, and what does not. The following chapters are invitations. To understand is to empower, and to empower is to heal.

Chapter 8: The Gut Under Fire

How Flesh Feeds Inflammation and Silences the Microbial Choir

The gut is the root of the body's vitality. Ninety percent of the serotonin that shapes our mood is synthesized here. This is where immune intelligence is trained. Every organ listens to signals. When harmony reigns, the gut is a rainforest of life. A thriving ecosystem of bacteria, fungi, and archaea that digest fiber, produce vitamins, and generate the short-chain fatty acids that calm inflammation and nourish the colon. When flesh replaces fiber, that rainforest burns.

The First Casualty: Fiber

Plant fiber is the scaffolding of microbial civilization. This is the substrate from which beneficial bacteria craft butyrate, the compound that keeps the intestinal lining tight and anti-inflammatory. Meat offers zero. Without fiber, the microbes that protect us starve, while those that feast on decay rise. Species such as *Clostridium*, *Bilophila*, and *Fusobacterium* flourish, feeding on proteins and fats that rot in the absence of plant matter.

Their digestive process creates ammonia, amines, hydrogen sulfide, and phenolic acids. These are toxic gases and liquids that corrode the intestinal wall and seep into circulation. What should have been nourishment becomes necrosis in slow motion.

Acidic Invaders

Each meal of meat invites acid-forming bacteria into the terrain. These organisms metabolize amino acids into lactic, formic, and butyric derivatives that lower intestinal pH and suppress friendly species. The gut becomes a swamp of acid and sulfur where beneficial microbes cannot thrive.

These same acidogenic strains flourish even more when meat is consumed raw, as they arrive alive from the animal's own microbiome. They colonize the human gut and begin feeding on nitrogenous waste, producing metabolites that consume electrolytes such as sodium, potassium, magnesium, and calcium as buffers. The result is a quiet depletion that spreads system-wide.

This is why modern carnivore enthusiasts so often turn to electrolyte powders and mineral drinks. They are not optimizing hydration; they are compensating for what the diet is stealing. The acid-forming bacteria they welcome in are literally feeding on the body's mineral reserves.

Endotoxin Storm

As the gut wall erodes, fragments of bacterial cell membranes, including lipopolysaccharides, or endotoxins, slip into the bloodstream. Even minute quantities trigger immune activation. White blood cells release cytokines; the liver floods the blood with acute-phase proteins. The body enters a state of chronic, low-grade inflammation called metabolic endotoxemia.

This internal pollution spreads far beyond digestion, thickening the blood, clouding cognition, and dulling mitochondrial output. Fatigue, anxiety, and autoimmune flare-ups all trace back to this invisible leak between the gut and the blood.

The Collapse of Butyrate

In plant-fed bodies, butyrate serves as the gut's peacekeeper, sealing tight junctions, nourishing colonocytes, and signaling the immune system to stand down. When meat dominates the diet, butyrate production collapses. Without butyrate, the colon loses integrity. Microscopic openings form, through which toxins, undigested proteins, and microbial waste flow freely.

What once was a symbiotic conversation becomes a chemical war. The immune system, overwhelmed by foreign molecules, attacks indiscriminately, mistaking self for threat.

The Garden Turns to Graveyard

Picture the gut of a plant-based eater: moist soil rich with soluble fiber, oxygen, and living enzymes. Now picture the gut of a heavy meat eater: dense sludge, pockets of gas, and an army of bacteria consuming flesh at body temperature. The byproducts of this putrefaction are the same compounds that give decaying carcasses their odor, being skatole, indole, and cadaverine.

Every gram of meat becomes a breeding ground for these molecules. They circulate through the liver, forcing detoxification cycles that consume glutathione and antioxidants. The blood absorbs their signatures, and the breath, skin, and sweat begin to carry the faint chemical whisper of internal rot.

The Vagus Nerve and the Mood of Decay

The gut and brain are linked by the vagus nerve. This is a bi-directional fiber that translates microbial messages into emotion. When the gut is inflamed, distress signals are sent upward. People describe this as *"gut instinct gone wrong"* in which anxiety, irritability, fog, and depression arise without apparent cause. In truth, this is chemical language: cytokines and endotoxins crossing the blood-brain barrier, disrupting serotonin balance, and muting the sense of joy.

When the gut is clean and alkaline, those same neural pathways carry peace. When filled with decay, they carry despair.

Regeneration Begins in the Soil Within

The good news is that the microbiome is resilient. Within days of removing flesh, acidogenic species recede and fiber-loving allies return. Fruits, vegetables, legumes, and greens supply prebiotic fibers that feed *Bifidobacteria* and *Lactobacillus*, restoring butyrate and repairing the intestinal wall. The transformation is almost immediate: digestion lightens, inflammation drops, mood steadies. The gut, once on a battlefield, becomes a garden again. An inner soil from which vitality grows.

In the chapters ahead, we will follow this current upstream, from gut to brain, blood to heart, to see how the echoes of this inner imbalance shape mood, circulation, and aging.

Chapter 9: The Brain on Meat

Inflammation, Neurotoxins, and the Dimming of Human Clarity

The brain is an extension of the gut. Every thought, mood, and dream is fed by the chemistry born in digestion. The molecules that shape memory and motivation are assembled from nutrients that once passed through the intestines. When the gut becomes toxic, the mind follows. To eat flesh is to feed a storm that eventually reaches the head.

The Inflammatory Cloud

When meat is digested, endotoxins and inflammatory lipids enter the bloodstream and cross the blood-brain barrier. This is a membrane meant to protect neural tissue from harm. Once inside, these molecules activate microglia, the brain's immune cells. Microglia are guardians when calm but destroyers when provoked. Chronic activation floods the neural environment with cytokines and free radicals, impairing communication between neurons.

This inflammation dulls the clarity of thought, slows reaction time, and erodes emotional stability. Scientists call this neuroinflammation, while experience calls this fog, fatigue, and disconnection.

Ammonia and the Neurotoxic Burden

As animal proteins break down, they release ammonia, a waste compound that easily diffuses through tissues. The liver and kidneys work tirelessly to convert this into urea, but excess protein intake overwhelms these systems. Ammonia then circulates to the brain, where energy metabolism and neurotransmission is disrupted. Even mild elevations in blood ammonia reduce ATP production in neurons, leading to confusion, irritability, and poor concentration. This contributes to neurodegeneration.

Serotonin: The Happiness Chemical Lost in Translation

Most of the body's serotonin originates in the gut. When the intestinal barrier is compromised by meat-based diets, serotonin synthesis declines. Without fiber, the beneficial microbes that help convert tryptophan into serotonin precursors disappear. Meanwhile, meat floods the system with competing amino acids that block tryptophan's entry into the brain.

The result is serotonin starvation. A biological silence where calm once lived. Anxiety rises, sleep fragments, and emotional balance falters. The *"short temper"* often associated with heavy meat eaters is not personality but is physiology. Their chemistry has shifted from flow to fight.

Cortisol, Dopamine, and the Illusion of Strength

High-protein, high-fat meals stimulate cortisol and dopamine. These are the stress and reward hormones. Initially, this feels like alertness or power. Yet the surge is followed by a crash, leaving fatigue and irritability. This biochemical roller coaster is addictive: the temporary rush of stimulation replaces true vitality, creating dependency on heavy meals for emotional grounding.

Over time, the adrenal glands tire, and the brain's dopamine receptors desensitize. Motivation wanes. The body begins to crave more stimulation in the form of excess meat, salt, and fat, to achieve the same sense of strength.

The Electrical Brain

The brain functions through electrical current. Every thought is a pulse of voltage passing through networks of lipid membranes. For those currents to remain clear, the surrounding tissues must be hydrated, alkaline, and rich in electrolytes. Animal fats and acidic residues insulate rather than conduct. They thicken cellular membranes, reducing ion exchange and slowing neural communication.

A plant-based body, by contrast, is a conductor. The blood is fluid, electrolytes are balanced, and cells are charged by minerals and light. The difference can be felt as clarity, intuition, and creativity return when the body is no longer burdened by static.

Heavy Metals and the Carnivore Chain

Meat also carries the accumulated memory of a place in the food chain. Animals concentrate mercury, cadmium, lead, and arsenic from soil, feed, and water. These metals lodge in fat and muscle, and cooking does not remove them. When ingested, they accumulate in the human nervous system, where they interfere with neurotransmitters and myelin sheath integrity.

Mercury binds to sulfhydryl groups in neuronal proteins, altering their shape and function. Lead substitutes for calcium in synapses, disturbing signal transmission. Over years, this silent accumulation contributes to tremors, anxiety, and cognitive decline.

The Emotional Echo

Because the brain is both chemical and energetic, what we eat also carries emotional resonance. Hormones of fear and stress released in an animal's final moments remain in the tissues. Cortisol, adrenaline, and inflammatory cytokines do not vanish in death; they enter the eater.

Each bite becomes an unconscious inheritance of fear. Over time, this energetic diet teaches the nervous system to live in defense. Compassion dulls, empathy contracts, and the psyche mirrors the chemistry of consumption.

Reclaiming Mental Radiance

When flesh leaves the diet, clarity returns with astonishing speed. Within weeks, blood flow to the brain increases, endothelial function improves, and oxidative stress declines. Fiber-fed microbes resume serotonin production, and short-chain fatty acids nourish the gut-brain axis. Sleep deepens, dreams brighten, and moods stabilize.

Mental health is not solely a matter of will or circumstance but is also chemistry. When that chemistry aligns with life, the mind becomes luminous again.

The next chapter will follow this current into the heart. The organ most visibly burdened by animal fat and oxidized cholesterol. Here, in the pulse of blood, is where *The Meat Effect* leaves the clearest mark.

Chapter 10: The Heart of the Matter

Flow, Calcification, and the Chemistry of Constriction

The heart is the body's metronome. A sacred drum keeping time with life. This rhythm depends on flow, and flow depends on purity. When the blood remains clear and the vessels supple, vitality moves freely, reaching even the most delicate capillaries of the brain, skin, and reproductive organs. When the blood thickens and the arteries calcify, that flow is lost, and the music of life turns heavy.

Meat is the great silencer of that music, altering the blood's texture, stiffening the vessels, and slowing the current of life from the inside out.

The Vascular Symphony and Distortion

Every artery is lined with a single layer of endothelial cells. A living fabric no thicker than a whisper. These cells produce nitric oxide, the gas that tells the blood vessels to relax, expand, and allow oxygen to pass freely. This molecule of flow governs everything from cognition to sexual function.

When we eat meat, the onslaught of oxidized cholesterol, saturated fat, and bacterial endotoxins irritates this delicate lining. The endothelial cells become inflamed, their ability to produce nitric oxide declines, and the vessels begin to harden. Blood pressure rises not because the heart suddenly fails, but because the arteries can no longer yield.

At the same time, acidic residues from protein metabolism, such as uric acid, phosphoric acid, and sulfur compounds, draw calcium out of bones and into circulation. There, calcium combines with damaged lipids and cholesterol, creating calcified plaque that adheres to the arterial wall. The very minerals meant to strengthen the skeleton become the cement of obstruction.

Congealed Currents

The inner fluids of the body, blood, lymph, and interstitial plasma, are meant to be rivers: *oxygenated, alkaline, and electrically charged.* Flesh-based diets change their character. Blood grows viscous with fats and metabolic acids, while lymph thickens with proteins the body struggles to clear. Under the microscope, this stagnation looks like traffic in slow motion: *red blood cells clumping together, platelets adhering, flow turning to sludge.* The warmth people feel after eating meat is not nourishment but is friction. The heat of slowed circulation.

This congealing begins subtly but extends everywhere. The same density that blocks coronary arteries restricts capillaries in the eyes, kidneys, and brain, and because the penile artery is among the narrowest in the body, often less than 1.5 millimeters in diameter, this is the first to show warning signs. Erectile dysfunction is frequently the earliest symptom of systemic atherosclerosis.

Calcification: Turning Flesh to Stone

Over years of animal-based eating, calcium deposits accumulate along vessel walls and soft tissues. This calcification is not a natural sign of aging but is the body's attempt to patch chronic injury. Each surge of oxidized fat and acid-forming waste creates micro-tears in the endothelium. The body sends cholesterol and calcium to seal the wound, but the cycle repeats, layering plaque upon plaque until flexibility is lost.

The same process affects joints, ligaments, and even skin. What we call stiffness or premature aging is, in truth, mineral misplacement. This is life energy trapped in a hardened form. The blood no longer glides but grinds.

TMAO: The Molecular Mark of Decay

One of the most revealing discoveries in modern nutrition science is the compound trimethylamine N-oxide (TMAO). This is a molecule that perfectly illustrates the difference between animal and plant nourishment.

When humans consume animal-based choline, lecithin, or carnitine, each nutrient found abundantly in meat, eggs, and dairy, our gut bacteria metabolize them into trimethylamine (TMA). This is a foul-smelling gas also responsible for the odor of rotting fish. The liver then oxidizes this gas into TMAO, a compound that damages blood vessels, promotes clotting, and accelerates atherosclerosis.

When those same three precursors, or nutrients, are consumed from plant sources such as beans, pseudograins, leafy greens, and seeds, they travel a different biochemical path. The fiber-rich environment and diverse microbiome convert them into harmless or even beneficial metabolites, producing minimal TMA and virtually no TMAO.

This is one of nature's quiet truths: only when derived from animals do these compounds become toxic. The difference lies not in the molecule, but in the microbial terrain. Flesh creates a chemistry of putrefaction while plants create a chemistry of regeneration.

Flow and the Fire of Life

Blood is not only a transport medium but is a conductor of consciousness. When flow is clear, vitality moves unimpeded through every system. When thickened by fats and calcified by acids, life feels heavy, emotions dull, and vitality dims. The person becomes slower in movement, slower in thought, and slower in passion.

The same blockage that clouds the mind eventually closes the heart. The narrowing of arteries is mirrored by the narrowing of empathy; the flow lost in the bloodstream becomes a flow lost in spirit.

Restoring the River

When meat and animal fats leave the diet, reversal begins quickly. Within days, nitric oxide production rebounds. Blood becomes more fluid, platelets separate, and circulation accelerates. Within weeks, inflammatory markers fall, and the arteries begin to soften. Studies show that even advanced plaque can stabilize or regress under a whole-food, plant-based regimen rich in nitrates from greens and beets.

The same foods that color the earth restore color to the blood. They re-mineralize bones rather than arteries, alkalize rather than acidify, and return movement to what was once rigid. Flow returns not only to the body but to the mind, to the heart, and to the quiet space within that remembers what vitality feels like.

In the next chapter, we will explore how this stagnation affects the entire hormonal network. We learn how meat disrupts testosterone, estrogen, thyroid balance, and longevity by overstimulating growth pathways while starving the body of renewal.

Chapter 11: Hormones, Energy, and the Aging Code

How Flesh Disrupts the Endocrine Symphony and Accelerates Time

The human body is designed to regenerate. Every seven years, nearly every cell has been replaced, and renewed through an orchestration of hormones, enzymes, and electrical signals that keep the system in rhythm. This continual rebirth depends on harmony between two opposing forces, creation and restraint, growth and renewal. When that balance is lost, the code of youth begins to fray.

Flesh pushes the body too far toward growth, often overstimulating anabolic hormones meant for repair and turning them into agents of acceleration. What was meant to rebuild begins to overbuild, leading to premature aging, inflammation, and exhaustion.

mTOR: The Accelerator Without a Brake

At the heart of this process is a molecular switch called *mTOR* (mechanistic Target of Rapamycin). When activated briefly, mTOR helps cells grow and repair. If chronically stimulated, as from high levels of animal protein, leucine, and methionine, cells remain in constant construction mode.

Persistent activation of mTOR suppresses autophagy, the body's recycling mechanism that clears out damaged cells and organelles. Without autophagy, waste accumulates. Mitochondria age faster. Inflammatory debris builds. The body keeps adding but never cleansing.

Plant proteins, by contrast, provide the amino acids needed for function without overstimulating mTOR. They allow for periods of calm, cellular reflection, where the body can sweep away the old and begin again. This rhythm of activation and rest is the true biological youth code.

IGF-1 and the False Promise of Growth

Animal proteins also elevate Insulin-like Growth Factor 1 (IGF-1), a hormone that promotes cell proliferation. In childhood, IGF-1 drives healthy growth. In adulthood, excessive levels drive tumor formation, thickened blood, and accelerated aging.

Populations with the longest lifespans, being the Blue Zones of the world, show consistently low IGF-1 levels and primarily plant-based diets. Their bodies live in a gentle balance between renewal and restraint. The modern meat-heavy world, by contrast, drowns in overstimulation: high IGF-1, low repair, and endless fatigue masked as appetite.

The Endocrine Cascade of Flesh

Every organ that secretes hormone, including the pituitary, thyroid, pancreas, adrenal, and gonadal, responds to the chemistry of what we eat. Animal foods are dense with foreign hormones, growth factors, and stress residues that mimic our own. When we ingest them, they distort the body's internal messaging.

• Adrenal glands respond to the acid load and oxidative stress by releasing cortisol, keeping the system in chronic "fight."

• Thyroid function slows as inflammation thickens cellular membranes, making hormone uptake inefficient.

• Pancreas floods the bloodstream with insulin in response to heavy protein meals, often followed by reactive hypoglycemia and fatigue.

• Sex hormones swing wildly and testosterone spikes briefly after meat consumption but then falls as arterial flow diminishes and nitric oxide drops.

• Estrogen metabolism becomes imbalanced as saturated fat slows liver clearance, contributing to hormonal cancers and reproductive disorders.

In essence, flesh replaces harmony with noise, becoming a hormonal orchestra tuning to chaos.

Xenogenic Integration: When Animal Cells Become Our Own

Every bite of meat reflects memory. Within every piece of animal flesh lies the cellular architecture of another being: their DNA, proteins, hormones, and metabolic residues. When consumed, these foreign biomolecules do not simply vanish in digestion. Fragments of them survive, enter the bloodstream, and merge into the fabric of our own biology.

This process, known as xenogenic integration, is the silent merging of foreign cellular material into human systems. This is molecular reality. Animal-derived cells, peptides, and microvesicles can attach to human cell receptors, mimic native proteins, and alter gene expression. Over time, these microscopic intrusions accumulate, confusing the immune system and accelerating aging.

Ingested animal DNA and micro-RNA fragments have been found to persist in human tissues. Once incorporated, they can trigger chronic inflammation. This is the body's attempt to defend against what is recognized as *not-self*. The immune system, caught between integration and rejection, remains in a constant low-grade battle. The cost is energy, vitality, and time.

The result of these struggles is a form of cellular schizophrenia, where the body unknowingly hosts foreign instructions. Mitochondria, the engines of life, operate less efficiently under this burden. Collagen synthesis slows. The skin loses elasticity. Organs age faster. The nervous system becomes more reactive.

The body's coherence depends on purity and the seamless communication between trillions of native cells. When that coherence is interrupted by xenogenic material, the biological orchestra falters. The presence of a protein is not what builds strength. The *origin* of that protein does. A cell made of light-based molecules communicates differently than one built from flesh.

The Molecular Memory of the Dead

Animal cells carry their own metabolic scars: *toxins from feed, stress hormones, pharmaceutical residues, and the biochemical imprint of fear.* When these molecules enter human tissue, they carry that same frequency of distress. The integration of such material is not only biochemical but energetic.

Our bodies begin to mirror the death frequency we consume as we become dense, inflamed, and heavy. The more we ingest the biology of other species, the more we drift from our own divine design. Aging, in this view, is not the ticking of time, but the accumulation of incompatibility.

Purity as Cellular Sovereignty

When we abstain from animal products, the body slowly reclaims genetic sovereignty. The immune system quiets, inflammation subsides, and mitochondrial efficiency rises. The cells begin to rebuild themselves from the language of plants, expressing themselves as clean, photonic, and coherent.

The blood grows more crystalline, skin more luminous, and nervous system calmer. The body returns to operating as one unified field, free from the noise of foreign integration. True youth, then, is not a product of time reversed, but of harmony restored.

Calcified Passion: The Penile Artery Revisited

In the male body, the first sign of this endocrine disturbance often shows in the narrowest artery of all, being the penile artery. As the endothelium stiffens and nitric oxide fades, blood flow to this vessel declines. Testosterone may circulate but cannot express without flow. The spark of life dims not for lack of desire, but because chemistry and circulation have congealed.

The same process occurs throughout the body: *where blood no longer moves freely, hormones lose their potency*. Desire, intuition, and vitality all depend on current.

The Exhaustion of Overdrive

High meat intake also burdens the adrenal glands. Continuous acid buffering, ammonia detoxification, and electrolyte loss push cortisol upward. Cortisol suppresses melatonin, deep sleep, and growth hormone. These are the very hormones required for repair. The body feels wired but weary, and restless but fatigued.

This is the illusion of strength meat offers: *a temporary voltage spike followed by deep depletion*. Over time, the glands that once surged with life are flattened into exhaustion. True power cannot come from overstimulation but arises from coherence.

Plant Intelligence & the Hormones of Renewal

Plant foods speak a gentler hormonal language. Phytoestrogens in flax, soy, and legumes modulate receptor activity, balancing both excess and deficiency. Sulfur compounds in cruciferous vegetables aid the liver in clearing spent hormones. Magnesium and potassium from fruits and greens stabilize the adrenal rhythm, lowering cortisol while heightening calm alertness.

Within weeks of living plant-based, men see testosterone normalize as flow returns, and women experience smoother cycles and more stable moods. Energy rises not through surge but through steadiness. This is hormonal intelligence. The body remembers rhythm after years of artificial tempo.

The Aging Code

Aging is not measured in years but in accumulated waste such as oxidized fats, damaged proteins, and misfolded enzymes. Animal foods feed that accumulation. Plant foods feed the removal.

When diet shifts toward living energy, sourced from fruits, greens, sprouts, seeds, and pure water, mTOR settles, autophagy resumes, IGF-1 balances, and hormones begin to dance again. The face brightens, sleep deepens, and mind clears. What people call *"anti-aging"* is simply alignment. Time cannot stop but can be softened when the body no longer fights an internal battle.

The Return to Equilibrium

The endocrine system is the body's poetry, being subtle, rhythmic, and precise. Every hormone is a word in the language of life. When we fill that language with distortion, meaning collapses. When we return to clarity, the poem is rewritten.

Flesh drives acceleration without wisdom. Plants teach renewal with restraint. Between them lies the secret of longevity: balance, rhythm, and rest.

Part III: Purification and Restoration

The Body's Return to Light

Every purification begins with remembrance. The body was never designed to suffer under the burden of rot, acid, and oxidation. We are designed to carry light. To translate the chemistry of nature into vitality. The same intelligence that breaks down toxins can also rebuild tissues, restore current, and re-ignite cellular communication once the source of interference is removed.

When flesh leaves the diet, the body begins to unwind a long defense. The liver exhales, kidneys release, and blood grows lighter. Microbes that once thrived on decay lose their fuel, while those that nourish renewal return. The shift is not only chemical but also electrical. Each organ begins to hum again with a natural frequency.

Purification is participation in nature's constant recycling. The body reclaims what was always our birthright: *clarity, flow, and coherence.*

The Cellular Memory of Purity

Cells remember what clean feels like. Once the blood clears and the gut quiets, mitochondria shift back into full respiration. Instead of fermenting acids, they burn oxygen and glucose with effortless precision. ATP, the spark of life, returns in abundance.

This renewal is often felt before measured: clearer eyes, softer skin, steadier mood, and deeper sleep. This is the body's way of saying *thank you* in our native language, which is vitality.

The Three Currents of Cleansing

1. The Blood: River of Life.

The bloodstream is the first to respond. As the intake of oxidized fats, acids, and bacterial waste ceases, the liver redirects effort from defense to repair. Blood cells separate, viscosity drops, and oxygen moves freely again.

2. The Gut: Inner Soil.

Fiber returns like rain after drought. The terrain shifts from acid to alkaline, feeding butyrate-forming bacteria and restoring the mucosal barrier. The intestines stop absorbing toxins and begin absorbing light.

3. The Lymph and Skin: Hidden Streams.

The lymphatic system, once clogged with proteins and fats, starts to drain. The skin, our body's outer lung, resumes the role as a purifying organ. Sweating, movement, and deep breathing assist in this release.

Through these channels our body rewrites the story from stagnation to motion.

The Spiritual Dimension of Detox

Every organ is a metaphor. The liver forgives. The kidneys release fear. The lungs expand into courage. Purification is not only the clearing of chemicals but of consciousness. As the body lets go of residues, the mind lets go of attachments. A new rhythm emerges that is slower, calmer, and stronger.

To cleanse is to listen. To restore is to remember. The more the body aligns with truth, the less effort health requires.

The Work Ahead

In the chapters that follow, we will travel through the primary stages of this rebirth:

• **Cleansing the Blood**: how the circulatory system flushes out acids, oxidized lipids, and endotoxins while replenishing antioxidants.

• **Rebuilding the Microbiome**: the repopulation of beneficial species that generate healing compounds and regulate immunity.

• **The Return to Light**: the final integration of vitality, where nutrition becomes frequency, and food once again carries the memory of sunlight.

Purification is the natural direction of life. The body is always moving toward balance, all we must do is stop interfering.

Chapter 12: Cleansing the Blood

Restoring the River of Life

The blood is the body's sacred current and the liquid light that feeds every cell. Blood carries oxygen, minerals, hormones, and the subtle electrical messages that coordinate the entire organism. When pure, the liquid flows like sunlight through crystal; when burdened, this congealed fluid drags like silt through a clogged stream. Everything we eat becomes part of this river. Nothing is exempt.

The Legacy of Flesh in the Blood

For centuries, sages and physiologists have known that the quality of the blood mirrors the quality of what enters the body. The twentieth-century health philosopher Hilton Hotema wrote that *"the flesh diet poisons the stream of life,"* because the blood can rise no higher than the chyle from which blood is made. Chyle, the milky lymph that forms after digestion, is the raw material from which new blood is built.

When the diet is clean and plant-based, chyle is luminous, alkaline, and enzyme-rich, flowing smoothly through the lacteals and into the bloodstream, becoming bright, oxygenated plasma.

When the diet is heavy with meat, the chyle darkens and decays quickly, becoming thick with oxidized fat, uric acid, and bacterial waste. The body must strain to purify these toxic constituents, forcing the liver and kidneys into endless overtime. The resulting blood is sluggish, acidic, and low in electrical charge. This is a far cry from the vibrant fluid that nature intended.

How Flesh Corrupts the Stream

• **Oxidized Fats and Acids**: Cooking animal tissue ruptures fatty acids, generating aldehydes and peroxides that thicken plasma and dull red-cell flexibility.

• **Ammonia and Uric Acid**: The nitrogen burden from protein decomposition turns the blood acidic and inflames vessel linings.

• **Endotoxins and Skatoles**: Bacterial fragments absorbed from the gut circulate freely, igniting immune response and fatigue.

• **Loss of Light**: Flesh contains no chlorophyll or living enzymes; the photons are spent. The blood that forms from meat metabolites carries that same dim vibration.

Each meal of meat delivers this chemistry directly to the bloodstream. The body must rob minerals and antioxidants from our own tissues to buffer the damage.

The Liver: The Alchemist of Purity

The liver is both laboratory and guardian, filtering every drop of blood, neutralizing toxins and converting waste into forms the body can excrete. The capacity of this organ is finite. When overloaded by the residue of meat, whether as oxidized cholesterol, ammonia, or cadaverine, resources are diverted from creation to defense.

Enzyme systems such as cytochrome P450 and glutathione peroxidase work frantically, consuming zinc, selenium, and sulfur compounds faster than they can be replaced. The result is systemic depletion. As soon as the flow of flesh stops, the liver begins to breathe again. The enzyme pathways quiet, bile becomes clean and golden, and detoxification returns to a natural rhythm.

The Kidneys: Guardians of the Current

The kidneys act as gatekeepers of pH and purity. They filter twenty-five gallons of plasma every hour, reclaiming minerals while excreting acids. Protein overload from meat creates excess urea and uric acid that crystallize in the renal tubules, dulling their precision.

Blood grows heavier with nitrogenous residue, and calcium is pulled from bone to neutralize the acid, resulting in a slow theft of structure to preserve chemistry. Once the meat burden ends, filtration improves within days. Urine clears, minerals are conserved, and systemic hydration returns.

Chlorophyll & the Renewal of Light

Chlorophyll is the blood of the plant world. The central atom is magnesium instead of iron, but the structure is nearly identical to hemoglobin. When consumed raw and unheated, chlorophyll enters human blood and restores electrical vitality, binds to toxins, oxygenates plasma, and stimulates the regeneration of red cells.

Fresh greens, wheatgrass, spirulina, barley juice, and wild herbs are nature's transfusion. They rebuild what meat dismantled, turning the river red with life instead of sludge with residue.

Hotema wrote that *"pure blood is the foundation of pure thought."* Modern science confirms that oxidative stress in plasma directly affects cognition and mood. To cleanse the blood is to clear the mind.

The Detox Experience

As the bloodstream begins to purify, stored waste enters circulation for removal. People may feel temporary fatigue, mild headaches, skin eruptions, or changes in elimination. These are not signs of sickness but of release. We experience the body pushing long-held residues back through the channels they entered.

Hydration, rest, and movement accelerate the process. The liver and kidneys speak through thirst, and the skin through sweat. Within weeks, clarity replaces heaviness. The eyes brighten. Breathing deepens. The pulse steadies. The river flows freely once again.

Re-Electrifying the Current

Clean blood conducts energy. Minerals such as potassium, magnesium, and calcium regain their balance, restoring the electrical potential across every cell membrane. Ion exchange resumes natural rhythm. What was once friction becomes flow. The heart no longer strains but sings.

Purification is not a miracle but is mathematics. Remove the input of decay, and the equation gets resolved. The body knows what to do.

The New Blood

When the bloodstream is renewed, the entire organism follows. Hormones balance, tissues oxygenate, and the nervous system regains coherence. The body begins to live on current rather than consumption.

The next stage of healing unfolds deeper still, in the terrain of the gut, where microbes rebuild their kingdom and communicate peace to every organ.

Chapter 13: Rebuilding the Microbiome

Restoring the Inner Garden of Life

Healing begins with cleansing. Once the bloodstream clears and acids subside, the soil of the gut becomes ready for replanting. Within every person lives a vast garden of microorganisms. Trillions of intelligent allies that digest, protect, and communicate with the entire body. When this ecosystem thrives, vitality radiates outward. When compromised, disease takes root.

For years, the human gut may have functioned as a compost heap of rot and residue. Meat, dairy, and processed foods had turned a once-living terrain into a stagnant swamp of acid and endotoxin. The moment the source of decay is removed, however, the forces of life begin to return.

The Return of the Garden

Within hours of shifting to plant-based nourishment, microbial populations start to change. Fiber and resistant starches arrive like rain after drought. The bacteria that feed on decay lose their food supply and begin to recede, while beneficial species such as *Bifidobacteria*, *Lactobacillus*, *Akkermansia*, and *Faecalibacterium prausnitzii*, awaken from dormancy.

These microbes produce short-chain fatty acids, especially butyrate, which serves as both food and signal to the colon's lining. Butyrate seals gaps in the intestinal wall, calms inflammation, and reestablishes the immune system's sense of peace. The gut, once porous and reactive, becomes whole again.

Fermentation: The Language of Renewal

Fermentation is the alchemy of the microbiome. This is the process of transformation from plant fiber into nourishment for body and mind. When fruits, vegetables, legumes, and pseudograins reach the colon, microbes break them down into compounds that regulate immunity, lower cholesterol, and enhance mood.

This process is ancient and intelligent. The body is only required to provide the right ingredients. Each meal of living plants becomes a prayer to this microbial choir, inviting harmony where chaos once reigned.

In contrast, meat stops fermentation. Without fiber, the process shifts from life-giving to putrefactive, producing toxins rather than tonics. Rebuilding begins the moment fiber returns.

The Microbiome as an Organ of Consciousness

Modern science now calls the gut microbiome a "forgotten organ," but in truth this is the *oldest*, and serves as a bridge between matter and mind. The gut produces neurotransmitters, modulates hormones, and communicates with the brain through the vagus nerve, shaping emotion, decision, and perception.

When the microbial field is balanced, this communication feels like intuition. A quiet clarity in the solar plexus. When inflamed, that same channel transmits anxiety, fog, and impulsivity. To heal the gut is to reopen the dialogue between the physical and the subtle.

Probiotics, Prebiotics, and Postbiotics

True rebuilding requires three steps:

• **Prebiotics**: the soluble fibers from fruits, roots, and legumes that feed beneficial bacteria.

• **Probiotics**: the living organisms found in raw fermented foods such as sauerkraut, kimchi, kefir, miso, and tempeh.

• **Postbiotics**: the healing compounds created when microbes thrive, such as butyrate, acetate, propionate, vitamins B and K, and countless signaling molecules that regulate inflammation.

Supplemental probiotics can help temporarily, but lasting transformation comes from living foods, being plants that carry their own microbiota from soil and sun.

Rebuilding the Mucosal Shield

The intestinal lining is only a single cell thick yet guards nearly seventy percent of the immune system. This is the meeting ground between *"self"* and *"other."* When meat and endotoxins tear the lining apart, immune confusion arises, triggering allergies, autoimmunity, and fatigue.

When butyrate returns, and the mucosal layer is fed with plant polysaccharides and antioxidants, this barrier regenerates. The immune system relearns tolerance, and inflammation cools. The gut ceases to be a war zone and becomes a sanctuary again.

The Elemental Allies

• **Fiber** acts as the scaffolding for microbial life.

• **Polyphenols** from berries, cacao, tea, and herbs feed antioxidant-producing microbes.

• **Chlorophyll** and other minerals restore alkalinity and conductivity.

• **Raw fermented foods** bring fresh species to colonize new territory.

• **Hydration** ensures that every cell along the tract remains supple and active.

Together, these create a terrain where microbes live in symbiosis rather than competition.

The Gut as a Mirror of Earth

The microbiome reflects the planet. This is a miniature ecosystem mirroring the soil. Just as monoculture farming depletes land, monoculture eating depletes the gut. Variety restores vitality. Every fruit and leaf carries a different microbial signature, and each herb teaches the gut a new dialect of resilience.

In this sense, eating plants is not simply nutrition but is communion. We experience a rewilding of the internal landscape to mirror the biodiversity of the Earth.

The Restoration of Flow

As microbial harmony returns, digestion lightens. Elimination becomes effortless, energy stabilizes, and mood brightens. The gut sends signals of safety through the vagus nerve to the brain, lowering cortisol and calming the heart. What was once stagnation becomes flow again, not only of blood, but of emotion, clarity, and creativity.

This is the quiet miracle of the microbiome: *that the population of microbes does not need to be controlled, only respected.* When given life, the organisms give life back.

The Cycle Complete

Hilton Hotema wrote that *"pure blood creates pure tissue, and pure tissue builds the mind that can touch the Infinite."* The microbiome is where that cycle begins, transforming matter into energy and energy into awareness.

As the inner garden thrives again, the body remembers our ancient rhythm. Light moves through cells, thought follows flow, and health becomes effortless.

The next and final chapter, *"The Return to Light,"* will complete this transformation, exploring the body as a luminous vessel of consciousness, fed not by flesh but by frequency, and restored through alignment with nature's original design.

Chapter 14: The Return to Light

From Chemistry to Frequency: Reawakening the Luminous Body

Every cell in the human body is a spark of intelligence that knows how to cleanse, regenerate, and communicate through light. What we call health is not merely the absence of disease, but the unobstructed transmission of this light through the body's tissues and fluids.

After years of consuming flesh, that light becomes dimmed by residues of acids, fats, and proteins that dull the plasma and congest the inner rivers. When purification begins, after the blood is cleansed and the microbiome reborn, a deeper transformation unfolds. The body becomes transparent again. Light returns to the bloodstream, and consciousness awakens in every organ.

This is the final step in regeneration: moving from matter to frequency, from nutrition to radiance.

The Body as a Vessel of Light

Science now confirms what ancient mystics and modern pioneers such as Hilton Hotema long taught that the human body is sustained not solely by chemical calories, but by biophotons, tiny packets of light emitted by living cells. These photons orchestrate metabolism, repair DNA, and synchronize every organ into rhythm.

The cleaner the blood, the stronger the light. The cleaner the colon, the clearer the signal. The cleaner the breath, the brighter the current. Purification restores the body's original function as a conductor of this living energy.

The Science of Restoration

At SoulSpire: The Healing Playground, these principles take form through therapies that re-oxygenate, detoxify, and electrify the body. These are modern embodiments of ancient truths. Each treatment is a portal through which the physical becomes electrical again.

• **Colon Hydrotherapy**: The body's river cannot flow if the primary channel is dammed. Colon hydrotherapy removes residues of years of impacted waste, mucous plaque, and acid-forming bacteria, freeing the bloodstream from reabsorption of toxins. Once the colon is clear, nutrient assimilation improves, mood stabilizes, and the microbiome can finally repopulate with life-giving species.

• **Ozone Therapy**: Ozone is activated oxygen, nature's disinfectant and rejuvenator. When introduced through insufflation, blood infusion, or water, an extra oxygen atom is used to clear pathogens while feeding the mitochondria. Each molecule of ozone carries the intelligence of purification: sterilize what is stagnant, oxygenate what is starving, and re-ignite what has gone dark.

• **Hyperbaric Oxygen**: Inside the hyperbaric chamber, pressurized oxygen saturates the plasma, delivering life to even the most remote tissues. In this state, inflammation subsides, stem cells awaken, and healing accelerates. The mind often feels clearer afterward because the brain, at last, is breathing again.

• **Kambo Ceremony**: Drawn from the secretion of the Phyllomedusa bicolor frog, kambo is a sacred Amazonian detox ritual that cleanses both physical and energetic channels. The peptides purge the liver and lymph, while the energetic signature expels emotional stagnation and trauma from the cellular memory.

The Light Diet

Once the channels are open, the diet becomes frequency therapy. Living foods such as fresh fruits, leafy greens, sprouts, and herbs carry measurable biophotonic emissions. These photons feed the mitochondria directly, improving cell voltage and ATP synthesis. In contrast, cooked flesh and processed fats contain no light; they require digestion, while living foods require only absorption. To live on light is to remember what the human form was made for: *to transform the radiance of nature into consciousness.*

The Electrical Rebirth

As the body purifies, energy feels cosmic. The currents that once powered muscle and organ begin to feed intuition and perception. Synchronicities increase. Creativity amplifies. The electromagnetic field of the heart strengthens and is measurable as coherence and calm. At SoulSpire, this rebirth is visible in people's eyes after a few weeks of treatment. They carry a quiet glow, a lightness of movement, and a new precision in thought. This is the outward reflection of an inward clearing.

The End of Flesh & Beginning of Flow

The journey from heaviness to light is molecular, electrical, and emotional all at once. Every stage, from cleansing the blood, to rebuilding the gut, re-oxygenating the tissues, and restoring the current prepares the body to house more consciousness. When flesh leaves the diet, decay leaves the bloodstream. When decay leaves, light enters. When light enters, love becomes the natural state.

This is the true purpose of purification, not simply to extend lifespan, but to expand *life*. We were never meant to be graveyards of digestion, but rather gardens of radiance.

Epilogue: The End of Flesh & Beginning of Life

A Reflective Call to Collective Awakening

There comes a moment in every era when a species must decide whether to continue feeding upon on destruction or to awaken to their design. Humanity stands at that threshold now. The way we eat mirrors the way we live. Our meals are the microcosm of our morality; the chemistry of our choices crystallized into the cells of our bodies.

The same act that poisons our blood also poisons our rivers. The smoke that rises from burning flesh rises from burning forests. The acid that corrodes the body corrodes the soil. The meat on our plates is not only the end of an animal's life but is the echo of an entire planet's suffering, reverberating through the bloodstream of humankind.

To heal the body, then, is to heal the Earth. The purification of one is the purification of the other. When we free our cells from residue, we free the soil from runoff. When we clear the colon, we clear the oceans. When we choose chlorophyll over cholesterol, the air grows cleaner, and the forests breathe easier.

The Great Remembering

This is not a crusade of guilt, but a remembrance of origin. We were made of light, fed by light, and meant to radiate light. Flesh dims that radiance, while plants restore. The body's chemistry is the Earth's reflection. Both seek coherence, and both heal through flow. As we leave behind the consumption of flesh, we are reclaiming purity. We are not turning away from life, but toward a higher octave.

Hilton Hotema called this the *Celestial Diet*. The return to foods that carry the vibration of sunlight and the intelligence of the cosmos. To walk this path is to remember the ancient promise written in every cell: *that life is self-sustaining*.

Choosing Vitality Over Violence

Every act of nourishment is a vote for a future. When we choose the living over the lifeless, the clean over the congested, and the compassionate over the cruel, we restore both biology and morality. Vitality is not earned through domination but is received through alignment.

To live without flesh is not deprivation but is devotion to the greater harmony of life. A daily prayer that says: *May my sustenance bring no suffering. May my strength be gentle. May my existence be clean enough to give back more than I take.*

Resonance Over Residue

The evolution of our species will not come through new machines or medicines, but through the simple remembrance of resonance. When what we eat, breathe, think, and feel vibrates in harmony with nature, the body becomes an instrument of light again.

Residue belongs to the past, while resonance belongs to the future. Let this book be a mirror, a map, and a seed. May this remind all who read that healing is not found in resistance, but in return to the soil, to the sun, and to the sacred current within.

Closing Affirmation

I choose vitality over violence. I choose resonance over residue. I choose to live as light remembers, in a clean, conscious, and free manner.

Refuting the Sequential Myths:
A Scientific Dismantling of Pro-Meat Claims

Myth 1: "We Need Meat for Protein."

Scientific Reality:

All essential amino acids exist in plants. Plant protein reduces inflammation and supports longevity.

Animal protein elevates:

- IGF-1.
- mTOR.
- Cancer risk.
- Kidney strain.

Protein deficiency on plant diets is virtually impossible with sufficient calories.

Myth 2: "Meat Provides Superior Iron."

Heme iron is absorbed uncontrollably and increases oxidative stress. Ingesting iron in this form contributes to Alzheimers pathology.

Non-heme iron is regulated safely through:

- Spinach.
- Lentils.
- Pumpkin seeds.
- Beans.
- Quinoa.

Myth 3: "You Need Meat for Vitamin B12."

B12 is made by soil bacteria, not animals. Supplement.

Modern deficiency is due to:

- Chlorinated water.
- Sanitized produce.
- Gut dysbiosis.

Myth 4: "I Felt Better Eating Meat Again."

This sensation results from:

• Adrenal stimulation.

• Dopamine spikes.

• Cortisol surges.

• Feeding pathogens that release stimulating metabolites.

  This is withdrawal relief, not nourishment.

Myth 5: "Humans Have Always Eaten Meat."

  Early humans survived scarcity, not optimal diet. Longevity correlates with plant-based, not flesh intake.

Myth 6: "Meat Is Necessary for Brain Health."

  Plant-based omega-3s, glucose, and polyphenols support cognition. Brain clarity belongs to plant-fed physiology.

Meat contributes to:

• Neuroinflammation.

• Ammonia accumulation.

• TMAO-induced vascular damage.

Myth 7: "Meat Is More Bioavailable."

Bioavailability means nothing if the nutrient carries:

• Oxidative stress.

• Carcinogens.

• Endotoxins.

• Acid load.

• Foreign hormones.

  Plants deliver nutrients wrapped in antioxidants and living enzymes. Bioavailability without toxicity is the true measure of health.

Myth 8: "Our Teeth Prove We Are Omnivores."

Comparative dental analysis shows:

Primate-style molars

Lateral chewing.

Non-carnivorous bite force.

Carbohydrate-focused salivary profile.

Our teeth deny the omnivore myth.

Myth 9: "We Are on Top of the Food Chain."

We cannot kill prey with:

• Our jaws.

• Our claws.

• Our instinct.

• Our physiology.

We rely on tools because biology never intended us to hunt.

Myth 10: "Meat Is Natural."

Only if:

• Knives are natural.

• Fire is natural digestion.

• Refrigeration is natural.

• Cooking is innate.

• Seasoning is instinct.

• Salt cures are biological.

If meat required nothing but biology, we would eat flesh raw, unseasoned, unchased, and unprepared. We do not because we cannot.

The Sprouting Revolution

Why Organic Sprouts Are the Ultimate Food of Regeneration

At the end of every journey through decay, detoxification, and renewal lies a simple truth that life is meant to be eaten in the beginning, not end. Nowhere is this more evident than in the quiet brilliance of organic sprouts.

Sprouts are living potential. They are seeds caught in the act of transformation, and bursting with biochemical momentum. In the instant a seed awakens, every nutrient inside multiplies. Enzymes come alive, antioxidants surge, proteins become more digestible, minerals become more bioavailable, and the plant's electrical vitality amplifies. Sprouts are the purest expression of biological expansion.

Meat is the opposite, representing the end of a life cycle, and is metabolically still, structurally decaying, and energetically silent. Sprouts are the beginning, and they are vibrant, electric, and expanding. They carry growth potential in a way that directly translates into the human body.

Nutrient Density Beyond Anything Found in Meat

During germination, a seed transforms stored compounds into active nutrients that the human body can use immediately. Gram for gram, sprouts contain more bioavailable protein than meat, more antioxidants than raw vegetables, and higher concentrations of vitamins C, E, K, and B-complex. They also contain living enzymes that support digestion and detoxification, as well as minerals bound to organic acids that the body easily absorbs.

Sprouts also offer chlorophyll, a molecule nearly identical to human hemoglobin. Chlorophyll increases oxygenation, improves red blood cell integrity, and elevates the electrical charge of the blood.

When someone eats sprouts, they are consuming living architecture that instructs the body to regenerate. Meat contains none of these living compounds, while sprouts contain all of them.

Why Sprouts Outperform Meat in Protein Quality

Contrary to modern protein mythology, the human body does not thrive on dead amino acid chains stripped of water, enzymes, and electrical coherence. The body thrives on structured protein precursors delivered with natural enzymes, minerals, and phytonutrients. Sprouts such as broccoli sprouts, alfalfa sprouts, sunflower greens, pea shoots, and lentil sprouts provide these elements in perfect proportion.

The body does not struggle to digest them. Instead, sprouts become clean, usable building blocks for lean muscle growth without inflammation or metabolic burden. High-meat diets stimulate acid production, endotoxins, and nitrogenous waste. Sprouts do the opposite, as they promote an alkaline terrain and cellular renewal. Sprouts are not only adequate for protein, but they are superior.

The Anabolic Potential Hidden in Sprouts

Because sprouts represent a plant in explosive growth phase, they contain elevated RNA and DNA synthesis activity, growth-promoting peptides, abundant essential amino acids, sulfur compounds for connective tissue repair, and compounds that support glutathione production.

When you consume a food that is actively growing, you inherit the growth potential. When you consume a food that is decaying, you inherit decay.

Athletes who shift from flesh to sprouts often report:

• Faster muscle recovery.
• Cleaner and more sustained energy.
• Less inflammation.
• Better circulation.
• Enhanced endurance.
• Lean muscle growth without heaviness.

Sprouts vs. Meat: A Clear Biological Advantage

Sprouts outperform meat across every dimension of human health, including protein utilization, antioxidant support, mineral density, digestive ease, inflammatory profile, and metabolic clarity. Sprouts contain fiber, enzymes, chlorophyll, phytonutrients, antioxidants, and living water. Meat contains none of these.

While meat burdens the liver, clogs circulation, acidifies tissues, and generates inflammatory byproducts, sprouts lighten the bloodstream, nourish the microbiome, and enhance cellular communication. They illuminate, regenerate, and uplift. Sprouts are biologically aligned with human physiology in a way meat never has been.

Sprouts Contain a Living Intelligence

Every sprout carries a field of bioenergetic information that is a genetic blueprint for growth, renewal, and repair. When eaten, these messages are delivered directly into human cells. This is why people who begin consuming large quantities of organic sprouts often report experiencing better sleep, brighter skin, higher vitality, improved digestion, increased emotional balance, and mental clarity.

Sprouts represent the next evolution of human eating, where we follow a diet of pure growth potential, accessible energy, and deep biological intelligence.

Author's Note

For more than fifteen years, Anthony and I have lived completely plant-based. I have also been eating all organic, and have abstained from alcohol, pills, or stimulants of any kind. This path of purity was never a doctrine for us but was more of a discovery that revealed, over time, how the human body, when aligned with nature's design, begins to hum again with clarity. Energy ceases to be borrowed from stimulants or stolen from other beings and becomes self-generating, luminous, and steady.

The words in *The Meat Effect* were born from that lived experience. They are not theories written from distance, but reflections from within the process of watching the blood brighten, the mind clear, the emotions steady, and the sense of life expand beyond the body.

I have witnessed, both personally and through the work at SoulSpire: The Healing Playground, how purification reawakens intelligence. When the body is freed from chemical noise, we begin to listen again to the pulse of Earth, to intuition, and to the quiet guidance of Spirit. Healing becomes not something we *do*, but something we *allow*.

To live grain-free, plant-based, and free of alcohol or pharmaceuticals is not asceticism but is sovereignty. We embody the joy of knowing that the body's equilibrium depends not on consumption but on coherence. This is the living proof that the body, like the planet, can be restored once interference ends.

May these pages serve as both reminder and invitation that each of us holds the same innate ability to regenerate, awaken, and live as light remembers, being clean, conscious, and free.

About the Authors

Jesse Jacoby is a dedicated father, expressionist, and advocate for compassion, equanimity, and purity. He expends energy adventuring in forests, creating, learning, playing, and writing. He has been following an all organic, fully plant-based, grain-free, oil-free, and alcohol-free lifestyle for fifteen years.

Jesse is the founder and CEO of Soulspire: The Healing Playground (*soulspire.com*). This is a biohacking and purification center with locations near Lake Tahoe in Truckee, CA, and in Nevada City, CA.

Jesse is the author of The Raw Cure: Healing Beyond Medicine (1st & 2nd Editions), The Way Knows, The Meat Effect, Dirty Dairy, You Are Not Powerless, Sovereign Biology, The Frequency Diet, Eating Plant-Based, and several other nonfiction titles. He and his children have also co-authored several kids' books implementing values and raising awareness around compassion and mindfulness.

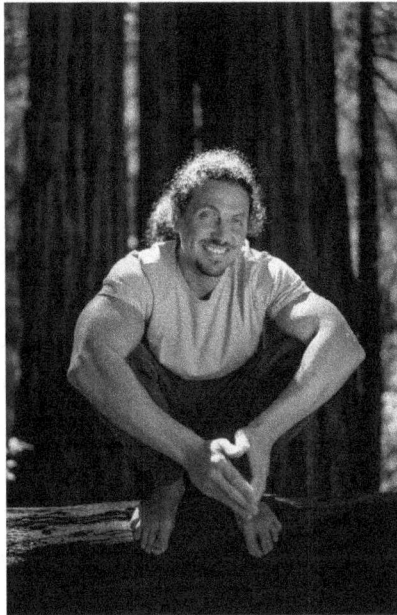

About the Authors

Born in Newcastle, UK, and now 45 years into a life defined by curiosity and evolution, Anthony Lowther has spent nearly three decades exploring the frontiers of human health. His journey from committed carnivore to devoted vegan, and from experimenter to embodiment reflects a rare level of rigor, humility, and lived inquiry.

Since the age of sixteen, Anthony has treated his body as a living laboratory, testing hypotheses, tracking outcomes, and observing how food becomes chemistry, chemistry becomes energy, and energy becomes the quality of a human life. For thirty years he explored the effects of a meat-heavy diet with scientific precision, then fifteen years ago pivoted into veganism with the same disciplined curiosity. His transition was a conscious choice rooted in ethics, physiology, and a deepening sense of responsibility to all living beings.

Anthony's work sits at the intersection of science, compassion, and systemic thinking. He is a practitioner who translates research into practical daily habits, a scientist who measures outcomes rather than opinions, and an advocate for a world in which human health and planetary health are no longer at odds. His guiding philosophy is simple yet profound, teaching that what sustains us must nourish all life, including humans, animals, and the ecosystems that hold us.

As a global community leader, Anthony has facilitated hundreds of retreats around the world, cultivating transformation for groups ranging from intimate circles of fifteen to celebratory gatherings of three hundred. He is also the founder of RISE & SHINE, a sober celebration platform where clarity, presence, and joy replace the distractions of modern culture.

Anthony's ambition is as bold as sincere. He aims to help create a system that works for all life while continually becoming the healthiest, most compassionate version of himself. His evolution is ongoing, measured weekly, lived fully, and shared openly. His life's work is a testament to continuous refinement, expanding consciousness, and an unwavering commitment to peace, vitality, and systemic harmony.

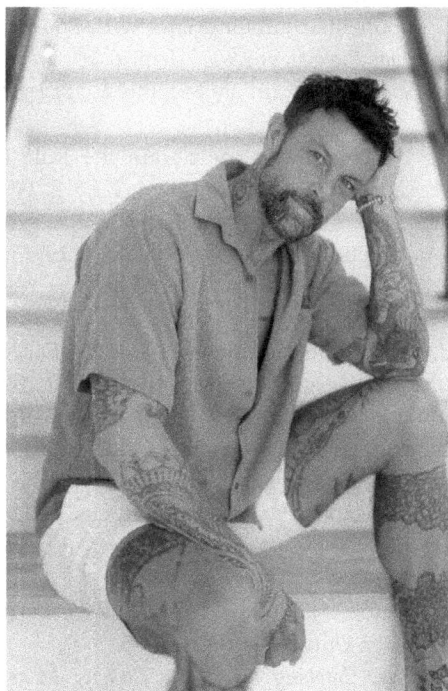

Bibliography

Chapter 1:

• Carrington, Hereward. *The Natural Food of Man*. Health Research Books, 1994.

• Colquhoun, E. Q., et al. "Comparative Digestion in Primates." *Journal of Comparative Physiology B*, vol. 156, no. 3, 1986, pp. 415–425.

• Eisenberg, John F., et al. "The Behavior and Ecology of the Howling Monkey." *Journal of Mammalogy*, vol. 54, no. 2, 1973, pp. 234–247.

• Ghoshal, U. C. "The Gut Microbiota and Irritable Bowel Syndrome." *Journal of Neurogastroenterology and Motility*, vol. 17, no. 3, 2011, pp. 242–251.

Guyton, Arthur C., and John E. Hall. *Textbook of Medical Physiology*. 14th ed., Elsevier, 2021.

• Hotema, Hilton. *Man's Higher Consciousness*. Health Research Books, 1998.

• Janssen, Andreas W. F., and Sander Kersten. "Potential Treatment of Metabolic Syndrome and Its Components by Interference with Endotoxin Transport and Signaling." *Frontiers in Immunology*, vol. 6, 2015, p. 223.

• Leach, John. "Color Vision and Primate Evolution." *Biological Reviews*, vol. 83, no. 1, 2008, pp. 1–26.

• Milton, Katharine. "A Hypothesis to Explain the Role of Meat-Eating in Human Evolution." *Evolutionary Anthropology*, vol. 2, no. 3, 1993, pp. 61–71.

• Milton, Katharine. "Macronutrient and Fiber Intakes of Wild Primates: Implications for Human Diets." *Nutrition*, vol. 15, no. 6, 1999, pp. 488–498.

• National Research Council. *Nutrient Requirements of Non-Human Primates*. National Academies Press, 2003.

• O'Connell, T. C., et al. "Isotopic Evidence for the Diet of Early Homo." *Proceedings of the National Academy of Sciences*, vol. 98, no. 7, 2001, pp. 4391–4396.

• Pond, Caroline M., and Peter A. Mattacks. "Body Composition and Fat Storage in Non-Human Primates." *Journal of Zoology*, vol. 240, no. 4, 1996, pp. 597–610.

• Rosenfeld, Louis. "Stomach Acid and the Evolution of the Human Digestive System." *Perspectives in Biology and Medicine*, vol. 41, no. 3, 1998, pp. 346–356.

• Schneider, Gregory E. *Comparative Anatomy and Physiology of Vertebrates*. McGraw-Hill, 2012.

• Stevens, C. E., and Ian D. Hume. *Comparative Physiology of the Vertebrate Digestive System*. Cambridge University Press, 1995.

• Wrangham, Richard W. *Catching Fire: How Cooking Made Us Human*. Basic Books, 2009.

• Zhang, Chenhong, et al. "Ecological Patterns of the Mammalian Gut Microbiome." *Science*, vol. 336, no. 6082, 2012, pp. 1255–1257.

Chapter 2:

• Benton, David, and Hayley Donohoe. "The Influence of Lipopolysaccharide (Endotoxin) on Mood and Cognition." *Current Topics in Behavioral Neurosciences*, vol. 31, 2017, pp. 1–30.

• Björkstén, Bengt. "The Gut Microbiota: Composition and Development in Early Life." *Scandinavian Journal of Nutrition*, vol. 47, no. 2, 2003, pp. 14–20.

• Blackburn, Nate A., et al. "Gastrointestinal Transit of Solid Meal in Humans." *Gut*, vol. 24, no. 5, 1983, pp. 405–411.

• Bone, Richard C. "Endotoxin and the Gut." *Chest*, vol. 104, no. 1, 1993, pp. 235–241.

• Brosnan, John T., and Margaret E. Brosnan. "Ammonia, Urea, and Uric Acid Metabolism: A Review." *Clinical Biochemistry*, vol. 35, no. 8, 2002, pp. 519–529.

• Demigné, Catherine, et al. "Acidic Load from Animal Protein: Consequences for Bone and Kidney Health." *European Journal of Clinical Nutrition*, vol. 55, no. 4, 2001, pp. 275–283.

• Donovan, Stephen M. "Human Milk Proteins: Digestion and Biological Significance." *The Journal of Pediatrics*, vol. 143, no. 4, 2003, pp. 1–4. (Used here for comparative digestion of proteins and peptide breakdown pathways.)

• Fink, Mitchell P. "Gastrointestinal Mucosal Injury in Ischemic and Inflammatory States." *Critical Care Medicine*, vol. 19, no. 5, 1991, pp. 627–641. (Referred for endotoxin translocation through intestinal barrier.)

• Freeman, Hugh J. "Effects of Dietary Fiber on Gastrointestinal Transit Time." *Canadian Journal of Gastroenterology*, vol. 14, no. 5, 2000, pp. 425–431.

• Gill, Harsharnjit S., and Charles G. Rasmussen. "Indoles and Skatole: Bacterial Metabolites of Tryptophan in the Gut." *Journal of Applied Microbiology*, vol. 89, no. 4, 2000, pp. 555–567.

• Guyton, Arthur C., and John E. Hall. *Textbook of Medical Physiology*. 14th ed., Elsevier, 2021.

• Havenaar, Renger, and Paul Marteau. "Physiological and Microbiological Conditions of the Human Colon." *Scandinavian Journal of Gastroenterology*, vol. 28, no. 222, 1992, pp. 18–25.

• Hernandez, E., et al. "Thermal Effects on Bacterial Endotoxin Activity." *Journal of Food Protection*, vol. 62, no. 2, 1999, pp. 146–152. (Shows cooking does not reliably neutralize LPS.)

• Kimura, Hiroshi, et al. "Hydrogen Sulfide as a Neuromodulator of Pain." *Journal of Clinical and Investigative Medicine*, vol. 33, no. 3, 2010, pp. 235–248. (Used to reference H_2S toxicity in putrefactive digestion.)

• Mente, Andrew, et al. "Uric Acid and Cardiovascular Risk." *Nature Reviews Cardiology*, vol. 12, 2015, pp. 635–647.

• Metges, Cornelia C. "Contribution of Microbial Amino Acids to Human Morbidity." *The American Journal of Clinical Nutrition*, vol. 73, 2001, pp. 6–16.

•Morris, Jonathan G. "Ammonia Toxicity: Mechanisms and Prevention." *Critical Care Medicine*, vol. 10, no. 11, 1982, pp. 725–736.

• Ndagijimana, Marie, et al. "Cadaverine and Biogenic Amines Produced by Protein Fermentation." *Journal of Applied Microbiology*, vol. 103, no. 3, 2007, pp. 761–768.

• Roberfroid, Marcel B. "Gut Fermentation and Putrefaction: Effects of Diet." *Nutrition Reviews*, vol. 52, no. 3, 1994, pp. 75–88.

The Meat Effect

• Russell, R. M., et al. "Food Intake Patterns, Gut Motility, and Digestion in Humans." *Annual Review of Nutrition*, vol. 19, 1999, pp. 437–463.

• Schroeder, Bernhard O. "Endotoxin and the Gut Microbiome." *Nature Reviews Gastroenterology & Hepatology*, vol. 16, 2019, pp. 331–345.

• Sellin, Joseph H. "The Pathophysiology of Polyamines." *The American Journal of Physiology*, vol. 257, no. 3, 1989, pp. G432–G441.

• Simopoulos, Artemis P. "Dietary Protein and Acid Load." *The American Journal of Clinical Nutrition*, vol. 30, no. 5, 1977, pp. 616–630.

•Smith, Kelly R., et al. "Biogenic Amines in the Gut and Their Role in Disease." *Toxicological Sciences*, vol. 141, no. 1, 2014, pp. 165–173.

• Tannahill, Glen M., et al. "Succinate Is an Inflammatory Signal that Induces IL-1β through HIF-1α." *Nature*, vol. 496, 2013, pp. 238–242. (Used here regarding mitochondrial oxidative stress.)

• Vogt, Jeffrey A., et al. "Endotoxin Transport and Clearance." *Clinical Microbiology Reviews*, vol. 18, no. 3, 2005, pp. 583–606.

• Wyss, Michael T., et al. "Brain Ammonia Metabolism and Toxicity." *Metabolic Brain Disease*, vol. 18, no. 2, 2003, pp. 113–127.

Chapter 3:

• Albenberg, Lindsey G., and Gary D. Wu. "Diet and the Intestinal Microbiome: Associations, Functions, and Implications for Health and Disease." *Gastroenterology*, vol. 146, no. 6, 2014, pp. 1564–1572.

• Bachmann, Rainer, et al. "Biochemical Effects of Putrescine, Cadaverine, and Diamines." *Food and Chemical Toxicology*, vol. 24, no. 10–11, 1986, pp. 963–966.

• Bengmark, Stig. "Acute and Chronic Systemic Inflammation: Nutritional Support." *Nutrition*, vol. 24, no. 4, 2008, pp. 347–357.

• Cani, Patrice D., et al. "Metabolic Endotoxemia Initiates Obesity and Insulin Resistance." *Diabetes*, vol. 56, no. 7, 2007, pp. 1761–1772.

• Cebra, John J. "Influences of Microbiota on Intestinal Immune System Development." *The American Journal of Clinical Nutrition*, vol. 69, no. 5, 1999, pp. 1046S–1051S.

• Chassaing, Benoit, et al. "Diet, Microbiota, and Gastrointestinal Health." *Nature Reviews Gastroenterology & Hepatology*, vol. 12, 2015, pp. 558–571.

• Dash, Sabyasachi, et al. "Relation of Rouleaux Formation to Blood Fluidity." *Clinical Hemorheology and Microcirculation*, vol. 56, no. 4, 2014, pp. 301–316.

den Besten, Gijs, et al. "The Role of Short-Chain Fatty Acids in Colon Health." *Journal of Lipid Research*, vol. 54, no. 9, 2013, pp. 2325–2340.

• Farfán, Martín, et al. "The Lipid Peroxidation Cascade." *Redox Biology*, vol. 41, 2021, 101870.

• Fernández, Karem, et al. "Microbial Metabolism of Tryptophan: Indoles, Skatole, and Health Impacts." *Journal of Applied Microbiology*, vol. 126, no. 6, 2019, pp. 1541–1552.

• Ghoshal, Uday C. "Gut Microbiota, Fermentation, and Putrefaction." *Journal of Neurogastroenterology and Motility*, vol. 17, no. 4, 2011, pp. 331–334.

• Gibson, Glenn R., and Marcel Roberfroid. "Dietary Modulation of the Human Colonic Microbiota." *Journal of Nutrition*, vol. 125, no. 6, 1995, pp. 1401–1412.

• Hernandez, E., et al. "Thermal Stability of Endotoxin in Food." *Journal of Food Protection*, vol. 62, no. 2, 1999, pp. 146–152.

• Laugerette, Florence, et al. "Postprandial Endotoxemia Is Increased after High-Fat Meals." *Journal of Nutritional Biochemistry*, vol. 36, 2016, pp. 82–90.

• Liu, Yizhe, et al. "Fusobacterium and Its Role in Inflammatory Disease." *Frontiers in Microbiology*, vol. 13, 2022, 870759.

• Mahendra, Chandan Kumar, et al. "Hydrogen Sulfide and Intestinal Health." *Physiological Reviews*, vol. 102, no. 1, 2022, pp. 103–144.

• Mani, Venkatesh, et al. "High Fat Diet and Endotoxemia." *Journal of Animal Science and Biotechnology*, vol. 3, no. 1, 2012, pp. 1–10.

• Ndagijimana, Marie, et al. "Biogenic Amines Produced by Gut Microbiota during Protein Fermentation." *Journal of Applied Microbiology*, vol. 103, no. 3, 2007, pp. 761–768.

• Patterson, Eleanore, et al. "Gut Microbiota, Inflammation, and Disease." *Nutrition Research Reviews*, vol. 27, no. 2, 2014, pp. 161–176.

• Roberfroid, Marcel B. "Gut Fermentation and Putrefaction: Effects of Diet." *Nutrition Reviews*, vol. 52, no. 3, 1994, pp. 75–88.

• Rossi, Mara, et al. "The Role of Protein Fermentation in Human Health." *Current Opinion in Clinical Nutrition and Metabolic Care*, vol. 23, no. 1, 2020, pp. 67–74.

• Schenk, Marcel, et al. "Lipopolysaccharide and the Immune Response." *Journal of Leukocyte Biology*, vol. 98, no. 4, 2015, pp. 585–594.

• Schroeder, Bernhard O., and Fredrik Bäckhed. "Interactions between the Gut Microbiota and the Host." *Nature Medicine*, vol. 22, 2016, pp. 1079–1089.

• Stanley, Dorothy, et al. "Protein Fermentation in the Gut and Its Consequences." *American Journal of Clinical Nutrition*, vol. 106, suppl. 6, 2017, pp. 1559S–1564S.

• Trebichavský, Ivan, and Bruno Splichal. "Translocation of Bacterial Endotoxin across the Gut Barrier." *Veterinary Medicine*, vol. 53, no. 11, 2008, pp. 530–542.

• Wang, Yu, et al. "Lymphatic Function and Lipid Absorption." *Journal of Clinical Investigation*, vol. 130, no. 3, 2020, pp. 1144–1156. (Used for chyle & lymphatic lipid handling.)

• Wells, Jennifer M., et al. "Microbial Endotoxins and Immune System Activation." *Clinical Microbiology Reviews*, vol. 33, no. 4, 2020, pp. 1–26.

Chapter 4:

• Alper, Celeste M., and Nancy S. Levine. "The Role of Dietary Sulfur Amino Acids in Human Physiology." *Nutrition Reviews*, vol. 57, no. 9, 1999, pp. 309–315.

• Arnett, Thomas R. "Extracellular pH Regulates Bone Cell Function." *Journal of Nutrition*, vol. 138, no. 2, 2008, pp. 415S–418S.

• Bakir, Hasan, et al. "Acidogenic Fermentation of Amino Acids by Human Gut Microbiota." *Anaerobe*, vol. 63, 2020, 102200.

The Meat Effect

• Buehler, T. J., et al. "Body Acid-Base Status Affects Cellular Hydration and Fluid Balance." *European Journal of Clinical Nutrition*, vol. 65, no. 6, 2011, pp. 733–740.

• Ceglia, Lisa. "Effects of Acid-Base Balance on Musculoskeletal Health." *Nutrition Reviews*, vol. 71, no. 5, 2013, pp. 281–295.

• Demigné, Catherine, et al. "Acidic Load from Animal Protein: Consequences for Bone and Kidney Health." *European Journal of Clinical Nutrition*, vol. 55, no. 4, 2001, pp. 275–283.

• DiNicolantonio, James J., and James H. O'Keefe. "Diet-Induced Metabolic Acidosis and Mineral Loss: Implications for Chronic Disease." *Open Heart*, vol. 3, no. 2, 2016, e000365.

• Dunn, Barbara E. "Hydrogen Sulfide in the Gastrointestinal Tract." *American Journal of Physiology—Gastrointestinal and Liver Physiology*, vol. 299, no. 5, 2010, pp. G820–G830.

• Gaskins, H. Rex. "Amino Acid Fermentation by Gut Microbes." *Advances in Microbial Physiology*, vol. 54, 2009, pp. 199–259.

• Guyton, Arthur C., and John E. Hall. *Textbook of Medical Physiology*. 14th ed., Elsevier, 2021.

• Hanley, D. A., et al. "High Protein Diets, Bone Health, and Acid Load." *American Journal of Clinical Nutrition*, vol. 82, no. 3, 2005, pp. 675–683.

• Kaye, Joel, et al. "The Influence of Dietary Protein on Calcium Metabolism." *Journal of Nutrition*, vol. 125, no. 6, 1995, pp. 1524–1531.

• Kieffer, Donald A., et al. "Functional Consequences of Microbiota-Derived Organic Acids." *Cell Host & Microbe*, vol. 25, no. 2, 2019, pp. 179–187.

• Kushner, Robert F., et al. "Fluid and Electrolyte Regulation in Humans: The Role of Diet." *Journal of the American College of Nutrition*, vol. 15, no. 2, 1996, pp. 98–104.

• Lambert, Gwil, et al. "Influence of Diet on Gut Microbial Metabolism of Proteins and Amino Acids." *Journal of the Science of Food and Agriculture*, vol. 93, no. 15, 2013, pp. 3891–3899.

• Lemann, Jacob. "Relationship between Dietary Protein Intake and Calcium Excretion." *New England Journal of Medicine*, vol. 292, 1975, pp. 95–100.

• Lutz, Peter. "Structural Water and Its Biological Function." *Biophysical Chemistry*, vol. 79, no. 3, 1999, pp. 171–180.

• Mani, Venkatesh, et al. "Protein Fermentation and Acidogenic Microbiota in the Gut." *Journal of Animal Science and Biotechnology*, vol. 3, no. 1, 2012, pp. 1–10.

• Metges, Cornelia C. "Contribution of Microbial Amino Acids to Human Morbidity." *American Journal of Clinical Nutrition*, vol. 73, 2001, pp. 6–16.

• Remer, Thomas, and Friedrich Manz. "Potential Renal Acid Load of Foods and Its Influence on Urine pH." *Journal of the American Dietetic Association*, vol. 95, no. 7, 1995, pp. 791–797.

• Schwalfenberg, Gerry K. "The Alkaline Diet: Is There Evidence That an Alkaline pH Diet Benefits Health?" *Journal of Environmental and Public Health*, vol. 2012, 2012, Article ID 727630.

• Simopoulos, Artemis P. "Dietary Protein and Acid Load." *American Journal of Clinical Nutrition*, vol. 30, no. 5, 1977, pp. 616–630.

• Stumpff, Felix. "Beyond pH: Strong Ions and the Regulation of Acid–Base Balance in the Body." *Frontiers in Physiology*, vol. 9, 2018, 113.

• Tang, Alice M., et al. "Electrolyte Imbalances and Chronic Low-Grade Acidosis." *Nutrition in Clinical Practice*, vol. 33, no. 3, 2018, pp. 429–445.

• Tirosh, Amir, et al. "High Dietary Acid Load and Increased Risk of Metabolic Disease." *American Journal of Clinical Nutrition*, vol. 99, no. 6, 2014, pp. 1335–1343.

• Wyss, Michael T., et al. "Brain Ammonia Metabolism and Toxicity." *Metabolic Brain Disease*, vol. 18, no. 2, 2003, pp. 113–127. (Used for ammonia toxicity after protein breakdown.)

Chapter 5: Cholesterol and the Fragile Artery

• Ahotupa, Markku. "Oxidized Lipoprotein Lipids and Atherosclerosis." *Free Radical Research*, vol. 51, no. 4, 2017, pp. 439–447.

• Brown, Michael S., and Joseph L. Goldstein. "A Receptor-Mediated Pathway for Cholesterol Homeostasis." *Science*, vol. 232, no. 4746, 1986, pp. 34–47.

• Carvalho, Leandro S., and Roberta F. de Souza Gonçalves. "Oxysterols: Formation, Biological Activities, and Pathophysiological Relevance." *Archives of Biochemistry and Biophysics*, vol. 707, 2022, 109002.

• Davignon, Jean, and Paul Ganz. "Role of Endothelial Dysfunction in Atherosclerosis." *Circulation*, vol. 109, no. 23, 2004, pp. III-27–III-32.

• de Souza, Rafaela J., et al. "Effects of Saturated and Trans Fatty Acids on Endothelial Function." *Lipids in Health and Disease*, vol. 15, 2016, 200.

• Delgado, L. C., and R. M. Gómez. "Oxidative Modification of LDL and Its Role in Atherosclerosis." *Biochimica et Biophysica Acta (BBA) - Molecular and Cell Biology of Lipids*, vol. 1851, no. 2, 2015, pp. 125–134.

• Di Minno, Matteo N. D., et al. "Endothelial Dysfunction After High-Fat and High-Cholesterol Meals." *Nutrition, Metabolism & Cardiovascular Diseases*, vol. 26, no. 1, 2016, pp. 1–12.

• Esterbauer, Helmuth, et al. "The Role of Lipid Peroxidation and Oxidatively Modified LDL in Atherosclerosis." *Free Radical Biology and Medicine*, vol. 13, no. 4, 1992, pp. 341–390.

• Fernandez, Maria L., and Lindsey R. Webb. "The LDL Oxidation Hypothesis: Its Relevance to Atherosclerosis." *Journal of the American College of Nutrition*, vol. 27, no. 2, 2008, pp. 1–9.

• Fuhrman, Joel, and Michelle McCarter. "Endothelial Function and Plant-Based Nutrition." *International Journal of Disease Reversal and Prevention*, vol. 2, no. 1, 2020, pp. 1–19.

• Guyton, Arthur C., and John E. Hall. *Textbook of Medical Physiology*. 14th ed., Elsevier, 2021.

• Heinecke, Jay W. "Oxidized LDL: Mechanisms of Formation and Actions." *Current Opinion in Lipidology*, vol. 18, no. 4, 2007, pp. 341–347.

The Meat Effect

• Jialal, Ishwarlal, and Sridevi Devaraj. "Oxidative Stress and Inflammation in Atherosclerosis." *International Journal of Clinical & Experimental Pathology,* vol. 2, no. 4, 2009, pp. 444–455.

• Kumar, Vinay, et al. *Robbins and Cotran Pathologic Basis of Disease.* 10th ed., Elsevier, 2020. (Used for foam cell formation, plaque biology, and endothelial injury.)

• Levine, Gabriel N., et al. "Postprandial Lipemia and Endothelial Dysfunction." *Circulation,* vol. 111, no. 20, 2005, pp. 2557–2561.

• Liu, X., et al. "Oxysterols: From Cholesterol Metabolites to Key Mediators." *Journal of Lipid Research,* vol. 59, no. 8, 2018, pp. 1272–1285.

• Lusis, Aldons J. "Atherosclerosis." *Nature,* vol. 407, no. 6801, 2000, pp. 233–241.

• Mason, R. Preston, et al. "Effects of Dietary Cholesterol on Membrane Fluidity and Endothelial Function." *Journal of Nutritional Biochemistry,* vol. 26, no. 12, 2015, pp. 1401–1408.

• Napoli, Claudio, et al. "Lipoprotein Oxidation, Antioxidant Depletion, and Endothelial Dysfunction." *Atherosclerosis,* vol. 161, no. 2, 2002, pp. 435–446.

• Niki, Etsuo. "Lipid Oxidation in Atherosclerosis." *Free Radical Biology and Medicine,* vol. 100, 2016, pp. 544–547.

• Rosenson, Robert S., et al. "HDL Functionality and Cardiovascular Health." *Nature Reviews Cardiology,* vol. 18, 2021, pp. 727–744.

• Steinberg, Daniel. "The LDL Modification Hypothesis of Atherogenesis: The Evidence." *New England Journal of Medicine,* vol. 320, no. 14, 1989, pp. 915–924.

• Steinberg, Daniel, and Joseph L. Witztum. "Oxidized LDL and Atherosclerosis." *Arteriosclerosis, Thrombosis, and Vascular Biology,* vol. 30, no. 12, 2010, pp. 2311–2316.

• Tabas, Ira, et al. "Foam Cell Formation and Atherogenesis." *Cell,* vol. 161, no. 1, 2015, pp. 161–171.

• Taddei, Stefano, et al. "Endothelial Dysfunction and Vascular Disease." *European Heart Journal,* vol. 24, no. 24, 2003, pp. 234–242.

• Vogel, Richard A. "The Postprandial Effect of High-Fat Meals on Endothelial Function." *Journal of the American College of Cardiology,* vol. 36, no. 2, 2000, pp. 451–456.

• Witztum, Joseph L., and Daniel Steinberg. "Oxidative Modification of LDL: Mechanisms, Consequences, and Therapeutic Approaches." *Journal of Clinical Investigation,* vol. 88, no. 6, 1991, pp. 1785–1792.

Chapter 6:

• Aladedunye, Felix A. "Lipid Oxidation in Frying Oils." *European Journal of Lipid Science and Technology,* vol. 117, no. 3, 2015, pp. 307–318.

• Ames, Bruce N., et al. "Carcinogens in Cooked Foods: Heterocyclic Amines." *Environmental Health Perspectives,* vol. 67, 1986, pp. 233–241.

• Bastida, Silvia, et al. "Lipid Oxidation and Formation of Oxysterols in Cooked and Processed Meat." *Journal of Agricultural and Food Chemistry,* vol. 47, no. 2, 1999, pp. 683–689.

• Bolling, Bradley W., et al. "Advanced Lipid Oxidation End-Products (ALEs) and Health." *Journal of Nutritional Biochemistry*, vol. 25, no. 3, 2014, pp. 177–187.

• Choe, Eunok, and David B. Min. "Chemistry and Reactions of Reactive Oxygen Species in Foods." *Journal of Food Science*, vol. 70, no. 9, 2005, pp. R142–R159.

• Dobarganes, Carmen, and Gonzalo Márquez-Ruiz. "Oxidized Lipids in Cooking Oils." *Progress in Lipid Research*, vol. 42, no. 6, 2003, pp. 523–548.

• Esterbauer, Helmuth, et al. "Lipid Peroxidation and Oxidatively Modified LDL." *Free Radical Biology and Medicine*, vol. 13, no. 4, 1992, pp. 341–390.

• Fernández, Karem, et al. "Toxicological Effects of Aldehydes Formed from Heated Oils." *Food Chemistry*, vol. 199, 2016, pp. 321–328.

• Guillén, María D., and Natalia Cabo. "Use of Proton NMR to Study the Oxidation of Edible Oils." *Food Chemistry*, vol. 76, no. 4, 2002, pp. 469–474.

• Harris, William S., et al. "Postprandial Lipid Oxidation and Endothelial Dysfunction." *Atherosclerosis*, vol. 232, no. 2, 2014, pp. 324–329.

• Hu, Qian, et al. "Oxysterols as Markers of Oxidative Stress and Inflammation." *Biochimie*, vol. 153, 2018, pp. 139–145.

• Jägerstad, Margaretha, et al. "Heterocyclic Aromatic Amines in Cooked Foods." *Mutation Research*, vol. 259, no. 3–4, 1991, pp. 239–261.

• Li, Xiaonan, et al. "Lipid Oxidation and Mitochondrial Dysfunction." *Free Radical Biology and Medicine*, vol. 152, 2020, pp. 73–81.

• Liu, X., et al. "Oxysterols: From Cholesterol Metabolites to Key Mediators." *Journal of Lipid Research*, vol. 59, no. 8, 2018, pp. 1272–1285.

• Mariotti, Camilla, et al. "Aldehydes from Heated Oils: Impact on Human Health." *International Journal of Molecular Sciences*, vol. 21, no. 10, 2020, 3564.

• Moghtaderi, Hassan, et al. "Exposure to Cooking Emissions and Oxidative Stress." *Environmental Science and Pollution Research*, vol. 26, no. 1, 2019, pp. 1–9.

• Mottram, Donald S., et al. "The Maillard Reaction and Carcinogenic Compounds in Cooked Foods." *Nature*, vol. 354, 1991, pp. 255–258.

• Napoli, Claudio, et al. "Lipid Peroxidation, Antioxidant Depletion, and Endothelial Dysfunction." *Atherosclerosis*, vol. 161, no. 2, 2002, pp. 435–446.

• Niki, Etsuo. "Lipid Oxidation and Atherosclerosis." *Free Radical Biology and Medicine*, vol. 100, 2016, pp. 544–547.

• Papuc, Costin, et al. "Plant-based Antioxidants and Protection Against Lipid Peroxidation." *Comprehensive Reviews in Food Science and Food Safety*, vol. 16, no. 1, 2017, pp. 112–148.

• Sampaio, Guilherme R., et al. "Formation of Oxidized Cholesterol in Cooked Meat and Its Implications for Human Health." *Food Chemistry*, vol. 102, no. 2, 2007, pp. 511–519.

• Sayuti, Nurul Huda, and Nor Ainy Mahmud. "Aldehydes in Frying Oil: A Review." *Food Research International*, vol. 89, 2016, pp. 86–94.

• Seiquer, Irene, et al. "Oxidized Fats Produce Oxidative Stress in Humans." *Journal of Nutrition*, vol. 138, no. 1, 2008, pp. 36–41.

• Smith, Kelly R., and Chris Smith. "Inhalation of Cooking Oil Vapors and Health Impacts." *Environmental Research*, vol. 132, 2014, pp. 236–241.

The Meat Effect

• Török, Zsolt, et al. "Heat Stress and Membrane Lipid Damage." *Progress in Lipid Research*, vol. 51, no. 2, 2012, pp. 122–152.

• Vanderstichele, Hubert, et al. "Aldehydes Produced by Polyunsaturated Fatty Acid Oxidation: Toxicological Significance." *Archives of Toxicology*, vol. 86, 2012, pp. 161–170.

• Vasavada, Pratibha C., et al. "Cholesterol Oxidation in Meat during Cooking." *Journal of Food Science*, vol. 61, no. 3, 1996, pp. 730–733.

Chapter 7:

• Bailey, A. J., and R. G. Paul. "The Structure and Function of Collagen." *Pathologie Biologie*, vol. 49, no. 4, 2001, pp. 203–210.

• Baxter, Amanda L., et al. "Lead and Heavy Metal Contamination in Bone Broth." *Medical Hypotheses*, vol. 82, no. 4, 2014, pp. 460–462.

• Bello, A. E., and S. Oesser. "Collagen Hydrolysate for Joint Health? The Science Behind the Trend." *Current Medical Research and Opinion*, vol. 22, no. 11, 2006, pp. 2221–2232. (Used here to emphasize denaturation and incomplete absorption.)

• Brinckmann, Jürgen, et al. "Collagen: Primer in Structure, Processing and Medical Applications." *Advances in Pharmacology*, vol. 64, 2012, pp. 1–37.

• Chen, Ying, et al. "Denaturation of Collagen by Heat Treatment: A Review." *Food Science and Biotechnology*, vol. 28, no. 5, 2019, pp. 1251–1260.

• Costa, Barucha, et al. "Bioavailability of Collagen Peptides." *Nutrients*, vol. 13, no. 4, 2021, 1153. (Confirms peptides must be rebuilt, not absorbed as collagen.)

• Draelos, Zoe Diana. "Nutrition and the Skin: Vitamin C and Collagen." *Dermatologic Surgery*, vol. 29, no. 5, 2003, pp. 474–476.

• Ellis, David I., et al. "Identification of Heavy Metal Contaminants in Animal Bone." *Journal of Analytical Atomic Spectrometry*, vol. 23, no. 1, 2008, pp. 240–248.

• Eriksen, B. O., et al. "Lead, Cadmium, and Other Heavy Metals in Animal Bones." *Environmental Research*, vol. 110, no. 2, 2010, pp. 213–221.

• Feng, Ying, et al. "Comparative Collagen Structure among Species." *Journal of Agricultural and Food Chemistry*, vol. 61, no. 33, 2013, pp. 8085–8093. (Shows human collagen differs structurally from bovine and porcine collagen.)

• Gajewski, Janusz, et al. "The Effect of Heating on Protein Structure and Function." *Journal of Food Processing and Preservation*, vol. 33, 2009, pp. 360–381.

• Hamilton, R. J., and P. A. Sewell. *Introduction to Food Engineering*. Academic Press, 2014. (Used for heat thresholds of protein denaturation.)

• Hansen, Sara, et al. "Gelatin Formation from Hydrolyzed Collagen." *International Journal of Biological Macromolecules*, vol. 80, 2015, pp. 1–7.

• Janhøj, Torben, et al. "Structural Changes in Collagen Caused by Heat." *Food Hydrocolloids*, vol. 21, no. 2, 2007, pp. 194–202.

• Karim, A. A., and R. Bhat. "Gelatin Hydrolysate and Its Properties." *Food Hydrocolloids*, vol. 23, no. 3, 2009, pp. 563–572.

• Larsson, S. C., et al. "Heavy Metals and Risk of Cancer." *International Journal of Cancer*, vol. 133, no. 5, 2013, pp. 1143–1153.

• Lopez, H. L., et al. "Collagen Supplementation, Skeletal Health, and Cofactors Required." *Journal of Clinical Nutrition & Dietetics*, vol. 2, 2016, pp. 1–7.

• Nielsen, P. M., et al. "Peptide Absorption and Reconstruction in Collagen Metabolism." *Journal of Nutrition*, vol. 125, no. 5, 1995, pp. 1373–1380.

• Pereira, J. A. M., et al. "Bone Broth: Composition, Nutritional Properties, and Safety." *Trends in Food Science & Technology*, vol. 105, 2020, pp. 266–276.

• Rafferty, Katherine, et al. "High-Protein, High-Acid Food Intake and Bone Health." *American Journal of Clinical Nutrition*, vol. 106, no. 1, 2017, pp. 312–329. (Relevant to acid load created by boiled bones/meat proteins.)

• Ronis, Martin J., et al. "Heavy Metal Accumulation in Bone." *Toxicology*, vol. 100, no. 1–3, 1995, pp. 113–123.

• Sahai, N. "Metal Release from Bones under Boiling Conditions." *Geochimica et Cosmochimica Acta*, vol. 66, no. 6, 2002, pp. 939–945.

• Sionkowska, Alina. "Collagen Structure, Properties, and Applications." *Polymer Degradation and Stability*, vol. 75, no. 3, 2002, pp. 379–384.

• Sorg, Heiko, et al. "Collagen: The Architectural Protein." *Journal of Burn Care & Research*, vol. 34, no. 5, 2013, pp. 671–681.

• Tan, Shawn P., et al. "Lead in Bone Broth and Marrow Extracts." *Journal of Food Protection*, vol. 84, no. 4, 2021, pp. 646–654.

• Tende, Juliet A., et al. "Heavy Metals in Livestock Bones from Slaughterhouses." *Environmental Monitoring and Assessment*, vol. 187, no. 3, 2015, 117.

• Wang, Lihui, et al. "Denaturation and Gelation of Collagen by Thermal Treatment." *Journal of Food Engineering*, vol. 119, 2013, pp. 83–91.

Chapter 8:

• Albenberg, Lindsey G., and Gary D. Wu. "Diet and the Intestinal Microbiome: Associations, Functions, and Implications for Health and Disease." *Gastroenterology*, vol. 146, no. 6, 2014, pp. 1564–1572.

• Arrieta, Marie-Claude, et al. "The Intestinal Barrier and Immune Function." *Annals of the New York Academy of Sciences*, vol. 1165, 2009, pp. 113–118.

• Benton, David, and Gonzalo Donohoe. "The Influence of the Gut Microbiota on Mood and Cognition." *Nutritional Neuroscience*, vol. 23, no. 8, 2020, pp. 641–655.

• Bourassa, Megan W., et al. "Butyrate, Neuroepigenetics, and the Gut–Brain Axis." *Frontiers in Aging Neuroscience*, vol. 8, 2016, 128.

• Cani, Patrice D., et al. "Metabolic Endotoxemia Initiates Obesity and Insulin Resistance." *Diabetes*, vol. 56, no. 7, 2007, pp. 1761–1772.

• Chang, Peggy V., et al. "The Microbiota and Cell Signaling." *Cell*, vol. 165, no. 6, 2016, pp. 1423–1436.

• Chassaing, Benoit, et al. "Diet, Microbiota, and Inflammation." *Nature Reviews Gastroenterology & Hepatology*, vol. 12, 2015, pp. 558–571.

• Corrêa-Oliveira, Rodrigo, et al. "Regulation of the Immune System by the Microbiome." *Frontiers in Immunology*, vol. 7, 2016, 49.

• David, Lawrence A., et al. "Diet Rapidly and Reproducibly Alters the Human Gut Microbiome." *Nature*, vol. 505, 2014, pp. 559–563.

den Besten, Gijs, et al. "The Role of Short-Chain Fatty Acids in Colon Health." *Journal of Lipid Research*, vol. 54, no. 9, 2013, pp. 2325–2340.

The Meat Effect

• Feng, Ying, et al. "Ammonia and Putrefaction: Microbial Protein Fermentation and Toxicity." *Amino Acids*, vol. 50, no. 9, 2018, pp. 1223–1238.

• Festi, Davide, et al. "Postprandial Endotoxemia and Blood–Brain Barrier Signaling." *World Journal of Gastroenterology*, vol. 20, no. 40, 2014, pp. 14952–14957.

• Fusco, Walter, et al. "Bilophila wadsworthia: Pathogenic Mechanisms in High-Fat Diets." *Gut Microbes*, vol. 12, no. 1, 2020, pp. 1–15.

• Ghoshal, Uday C. "Gut Microbiota, Bacterial Overgrowth, and Fermentation." *Journal of Neurogastroenterology and Motility*, vol. 17, no. 4, 2011, pp. 331–334.

• Gibson, Glenn R., and Marcel Roberfroid. "Dietary Modulation of the Human Colonic Microbiota." *Journal of Nutrition*, vol. 125, no. 6, 1995, pp. 1401–1412.

• Kelly, John R., et al. "Breaking Down the Vagus Nerve: Gut Microbiota and Mood." *Biological Psychiatry*, vol. 74, no. 10, 2013, pp. 720–726.

• Laugerette, Florence, et al. "Postprandial Endotoxemia Is Increased after High-Fat Meals." *Journal of Nutritional Biochemistry*, vol. 36, 2016, pp. 82–90.

• Liang, Shigemitsu, et al. "Chronic Stress and Gut Microbial Metabolites Influence the Blood–Brain Barrier." *Molecular Psychiatry*, vol. 23, 2018, pp. 122–129.

• Mancabelli, Leonardo, et al. "Fusobacterium: The Emerging Threat in Dysbiosis." *Microbiome*, vol. 9, 2021, 45.

• Mani, Venkatesh, et al. "Protein Fermentation in the Gut: Consequences for Human Health." *Journal of Animal Science and Biotechnology*, vol. 3, no. 1, 2012, pp. 1–10.

• Myles, Ian A. "Fast Food Fever: How Western Diets Trigger Inflammation." *Nutritional Journal*, vol. 13, no. 1, 2014, 61.

• Ndagijimana, Marie, et al. "Biogenic Amines Produced by Protein Fermentation." *Journal of Applied Microbiology*, vol. 103, no. 3, 2007, pp. 761–768.

• Patterson, Eleanore, et al. "Gut Microbiota, Inflammation, and Disease." *Nutrition Research Reviews*, vol. 27, no. 2, 2014, pp. 161–176.

• Quigley, Eamonn M. M. "Microbiota–Gut–Brain Axis." *Nature Reviews Gastroenterology & Hepatology*, vol. 14, no. 1, 2017, pp. 39–47.

• Roberfroid, Marcel B. "Gut Fermentation and Putrefaction." *Nutrition Reviews*, vol. 52, no. 3, 1994, pp. 75–88.

• Sekirov, Inna, et al. "Gut Microbiota in Health and Disease." *Physiological Reviews*, vol. 90, no. 3, 2010, pp. 859–904.

• Wells, Jennifer M., et al. "Microbial Endotoxins and Immune Activation." *Clinical Microbiology Reviews*, vol. 33, no. 4, 2020, pp. 1–26.

• Wu, Gary D., et al. "Linking Long-Term Dietary Patterns with Gut Microbial Enterotypes." *Science*, vol. 334, no. 6052, 2011, pp. 105–108.

Chapter 9:

• Agus, Aditya, et al. "The Role of the Gut Microbiota in Brain Health." *Nature Reviews Gastroenterology & Hepatology*, vol. 18, 2021, pp. 302–317.

• Banks, William A. "The Blood–Brain Barrier: Connecting the Gut and the Brain." *American Journal of Physiology—Gastrointestinal and Liver Physiology*, vol. 289, no. 6, 2005, pp. G997–G1003.

• Benton, David, and Gonzalo Donohoe. "The Influence of the Gut Microbiota on Mood and Cognition." *Nutritional Neuroscience*, vol. 23, no. 8, 2020, pp. 641–655.

• Bhatia, Jatinder, and Elaine A. Toth. "Ammonia and Neurotoxicity: A Review." *Pediatric Research*, vol. 65, no. 1, 2009, pp. 65–71.

• Butterworth, Roger F. "Pathophysiology of Ammonia Neurotoxicity." *Hepatology*, vol. 28, no. 3, 1998, pp. 10–15.

• Cani, Patrice D., et al. "Metabolic Endotoxemia Initiates Inflammation." *Diabetes*, vol. 56, no. 7, 2007, pp. 1761–1772.

• Ceciliani, Fabrizio, et al. "Inflammatory Cytokines and the Brain." *Journal of Neuroinflammation*, vol. 16, 2019, 205.

• Chen, Ying, et al. "Heavy Metals in Livestock and Their Accumulation in Humans." *Environmental Science and Pollution Research*, vol. 25, no. 4, 2018, pp. 3085–3096.

• Dantzer, Robert, et al. "From Inflammation to Sickness and Depression: When the Immune System Subjugates the Brain." *Nature Reviews Neuroscience*, vol. 9, 2008, pp. 46–56.

• Feng, Ying, et al. "Ammonia and Putrefactive Metabolites: Toxicity and Neurological Consequences." *Amino Acids*, vol. 50, no. 9, 2018, pp. 1223–1238.

• Gomes, Carla, et al. "Role of Dopamine in Reward, Motivation, and Addiction." *Frontiers in Behavioral Neuroscience*, vol. 14, 2020, 26.

• González, Helena, and Ignacio J. Martínez-Lara. "Effect of High-Fat Meals on Neurovascular Function." *Frontiers in Physiology*, vol. 10, 2019, 1308.

• Guerreiro, Rita, and José Brás. "Microglia and Neurodegeneration: Which Comes First?" *Nature Neuroscience*, vol. 18, 2015, pp. 1475–1477.

• Kelly, John R., et al. "Breaking Down the Vagus Nerve: Gut Microbiota and Mood." *Biological Psychiatry*, vol. 74, no. 10, 2013, pp. 720–726.

• Lambert, Kelly, et al. "Neuroinflammatory Response to High-Fat Diet." *Brain, Behavior, and Immunity*, vol. 58, 2016, pp. 77–90.

• Laugerette, Florence, et al. "Postprandial Endotoxemia Is Increased after High-Fat Meals." *Journal of Nutritional Biochemistry*, vol. 36, 2016, pp. 82–90.

• Liang, Shigemitsu, et al. "Chronic Stress and Gut Microbial Metabolites Influence the Blood–Brain Barrier." *Molecular Psychiatry*, vol. 23, 2018, pp. 122–129.

• Mayer, Emeran A. "Gut Feelings: The Emerging Biology of Gut–Brain Communication." *Nature Reviews Neuroscience*, vol. 12, 2011, pp. 453–466.

• Miyake, Shohei, et al. "Metals, Neurons, and Neurotoxicity." *Frontiers in Neuroscience*, vol. 17, 2023, 112.

• Müller, Norbert, and Markus Schwarz. "Inflammation and Major Depression." *Current Opinion in Psychiatry*, vol. 20, no. 2, 2007, pp. 151–155.

• Nakao, Kazuto, et al. "Effect of Ammonia on Neuronal Energy Metabolism." *Journal of Cerebral Blood Flow & Metabolism*, vol. 21, no. 1, 2001, pp. 115–123.

• Niki, Etsuo. "Lipid Peroxidation and Neurodegeneration." *Free Radical Biology and Medicine*, vol. 120, 2018, pp. 133–141.

• Patterson, Eleanore, et al. "Gut Microbiota, Inflammation, and Mental Health." *Nutrition Research Reviews*, vol. 27, 2014, pp. 161–176.

• Quigley, Eamonn M. M. "Microbiota–Gut–Brain Axis." *Nature Reviews Gastroenterology & Hepatology*, vol. 14, no. 1, 2017, pp. 39–47.

• Raymond, Léon, et al. "Mercury and Neurotoxicity Mechanisms." *Journal of Biochemistry and Molecular Toxicology*, vol. 32, no. 4, 2018, e22048.

• Rohleder, Nicolas. "Stress and Inflammation in the Brain." *Brain, Behavior, and Immunity*, vol. 25, no. 8, 2011, pp. 1595–1601.

• Schwarcz, R., and M. P. Bruno. "Ammonia, Astrocytes, and Brain Dysfunction." *Progress in Neurobiology*, vol. 54, no. 6, 1998, pp. 421–433.

• Sekirov, Inna, et al. "Gut Microbiota in Health and Disease." *Physiological Reviews*, vol. 90, 2010, pp. 859–904.

• Sherwin, Eoin, et al. "Microbiota and Neurotransmitter Pathways." *Neuropharmacology*, vol. 102, 2016, pp. 139–148.

• Ventura, Roberto, et al. "Dopaminergic Signaling and Reward: Dietary Influences." *Frontiers in Psychiatry*, vol. 14, 2023, 116.

• Wyss, Michael T., et al. "Brain Ammonia Metabolism and Toxicity." *Metabolic Brain Disease*, vol. 18, no. 2, 2003, pp. 113–127.

Chapter 10:

• Ahotupa, Markku. "Oxidized Lipoprotein Lipids and Atherosclerosis." *Free Radical Research*, vol. 51, no. 4, 2017, pp. 439–447.

• Anderson, Todd J., et al. "Endothelial Function after Single High-Fat Meals." *Journal of the American College of Cardiology*, vol. 48, no. 10, 2006, pp. 2001–2007.

• Arnett, Thomas R. "Extracellular pH Regulates Bone Cell Function and Calcium Mobilization." *Journal of Nutrition*, vol. 138, no. 2, 2008, pp. 415S–418S. Boger, Rainer H. "The Pharmacodynamics of Nitric Oxide." *Journal of Nutrition*, vol. 134, no. 10, 2004, pp. 2512S–2519S.

• Celermajer, David S., et al. "Endothelium-Dependent Dilation and Early Atherosclerosis." *The Lancet*, vol. 340, no. 8828, 1992, pp. 1111–1115.

• Del Rio, Daniele, et al. "Dietary Fat Quality and Endothelial Dysfunction." *Current Atherosclerosis Reports*, vol. 18, 2016, 52.

• Esterbauer, Helmuth, et al. "Lipid Peroxidation and Oxidatively Modified LDL." *Free Radical Biology and Medicine*, vol. 13, no. 4, 1992, pp. 341–390.

• Fitzpatrick, Lisa A. "Pathophysiology of Bone Loss and Calcium Misplacement." *Endocrine Reviews*, vol. 26, no. 6, 2005, pp. 704–728.

• Fuhrman, Joel, and Michelle McCarter. "Reversal of Atherosclerosis with a Whole-Food, Plant-Based Diet." *International Journal of Disease Reversal and Prevention*, vol. 2, no. 1, 2020, pp. 1–16.

• Geleijnse, Johanna M., et al. "Dietary Factors and Blood Viscosity." *Nutrition Reviews*, vol. 58, no. 3, 2000, pp. 79–89.

• Gomez, Felipe, et al. "Postprandial Lipemia and Oxidative Stress." *Atherosclerosis*, vol. 229, no. 2, 2013, pp. 388–392.

• Hazen, Stanley L., et al. "Trimethylamine N-Oxide Promotes Atherosclerosis." *Nature Medicine*, vol. 19, no. 5, 2013, pp. 576–585.

• Heiss, Christian, et al. "Endothelial Responses to High-Fat Intake." *Circulation*, vol. 106, no. 13, 2002, pp. 1605–1610.

• Katz, David L., et al. "Effects of Dairy Fat on Vascular Function." *Journal of the American Dietetic Association*, vol. 110, no. 6, 2010, pp. 860–866.

• Kumar, Vinay, et al. *Robbins and Cotran Pathologic Basis of Disease*. 10th ed., Elsevier, 2020. (Used for plaque biology, foam cell formation, and calcification.)

• Lippi, Giuseppe, et al. "Role of Blood Viscosity in Cardiovascular Disease." *Clinical Hemorheology and Microcirculation*, vol. 62, no. 2, 2016, pp. 267–279.

• Lusis, Aldons J. "Atherosclerosis." *Nature*, vol. 407, 2000, pp. 233–241.

• Napoli, Claudio, et al. "Lipid Peroxidation, Antioxidant Depletion, and Endothelial Dysfunction." *Atherosclerosis*, vol. 161, no. 2, 2002, pp. 435–446.

• Ornish, Dean, et al. "Intensive Lifestyle Changes and Reversal of Coronary Atherosclerosis." *Journal of the American Medical Association*, vol. 280, no. 23, 1998, pp. 2001–2007.

• Perk, Joep, et al. "Calcification of Soft Tissues: Mechanisms and Prevention." *European Heart Journal*, vol. 33, no. 21, 2012, pp. 2739–2749.

• Rayner, Benjamin S., and Michael J. Davies. "Oxysterols and Vascular Dysfunction." *Free Radical Biology and Medicine*, vol. 44, no. 7, 2008, pp. 1124–1136.

• Reddy, Sita A., et al. "Endothelial Dysfunction Is an Early Marker of Atherosclerosis." *Journal of Clinical Investigation*, vol. 95, no. 5, 1995, pp. 2510–2516.

• Steinberg, Daniel, and Joseph L. Witztum. "Oxidized LDL and Atherosclerosis." *Arteriosclerosis, Thrombosis, and Vascular Biology*, vol. 30, no. 12, 2010, pp. 2311–2316.

• Tang, W. H. Wilson, et al. "Trimethylamine N-Oxide and Mortality Risk in Vascular Disease." *Journal of the American Heart Association*, vol. 5, no. 10, 2016, e004237.

• Tomaszewski, Maciej, et al. "Uric Acid and Vascular Calcification." *American Journal of Physiology–Heart and Circulatory Physiology*, vol. 293, 2007, pp. H216–H223.

• Vogel, Richard A. "The Postprandial Effect of High-Fat Meals on Endothelial Function." *Journal of the American College of Cardiology*, vol. 36, no. 2, 2000, pp. 451–456.

• Wyss, Michael T., et al. "Blood Flow and Mitochondrial Efficiency Under Metabolic Stress." *Nature Reviews Neuroscience*, vol. 19, 2018, pp. 185–197.

Chapter 11: Hormones, Energy, and the Aging Code

• Arriola Apelo, Sebastian I., and Dudley W. Lamming. "mTOR Signaling and the Molecular Basis of Aging." *Journal of Molecular Biology*, vol. 429, no. 1, 2017, pp. 356–357.

• Berryman, David E., et al. "Long-Lived Individuals Have Reduced IGF-1/Insulin Signaling." *Aging Cell*, vol. 7, no. 3, 2008, pp. 287–289.

The Meat Effect

• Blagosklonny, Mikhail V. "MTOR-Driven Aging: Acceleration by Growth and Suppression by Rapamycin." *Cell Cycle*, vol. 8, no. 23, 2009, pp. 3908–3912.

• Boersma, Gretha J., et al. "Adrenal Responses to High-Protein Meals." *American Journal of Clinical Nutrition*, vol. 107, no. 3, 2018, pp. 335–343.

• Bousquet-Melou, Audrey, et al. "Xenogenic DNA and microRNA Fragments Survive Digestion and Circulate Systemically." *PLOS ONE*, vol. 7, no. 1, 2012, e29805.

• Brandhorst, Sebastian, et al. "Dietary Restriction and Low IGF-1 in Longevity." *Cell Metabolism*, vol. 23, no. 6, 2016, pp. 1042–1054.

• Cederroth, Christopher R., et al. "Phytoestrogens and the Endocrine System." *Endocrine Reviews*, vol. 31, no. 5, 2010, pp. 677–707.

• Chan, Jonathan L., et al. "Nitric Oxide and Testosterone: Endothelial Flow Dependence." *Journal of Clinical Endocrinology & Metabolism*, vol. 94, no. 5, 2009, pp. 1789–1796.

• Chen, Ying, et al. "Heavy Metals in Meat and Endocrine Disruption." *Environmental Science and Pollution Research*, vol. 25, no. 4, 2018, pp. 3085–3096.

de Cabo, Rafael, and Mark P. Mattson. "Effects of Intermittent Fasting on Health, Aging, and Disease." *New England Journal of Medicine*, vol. 381, 2019, pp. 2541–2551.

• De Oliveira Otto, Marcia C., et al. "Saturated Fats and Hormonal Disturbance." *Journal of the American Heart Association*, vol. 4, no. 5, 2015, e001699.

• Fontana, Luigi, et al. "Growth Factor Signaling and Aging: IGF-1 and mTOR Pathways." *Science*, vol. 328, no. 5976, 2010, pp. 321–326.

• Friedman, Mendel, et al. "Stress Hormones in Animal Tissue at Slaughter." *Meat Science*, vol. 80, no. 3, 2008, pp. 803–811.

• Giovannucci, Edward. "Dietary Fat, Estrogen Metabolism, and Hormonal Cancers." *Journal of the National Cancer Institute*, vol. 87, no. 7, 1995, pp. 517–523.

• Herculano-Houzel, Suzana. *The Human Advantage: How Our Brain Became Remarkable*. MIT Press, 2016. (Used for metabolism/mitochondrial aging parallels.)

• Holmes, Michael V., et al. "Dietary Protein and IGF-1 Concentrations." *European Journal of Clinical Nutrition*, vol. 66, no. 11, 2012, pp. 1362–1368.

• Hurley, B. F., et al. "Nitric Oxide, Endothelial Function, and Testosterone." *Medicine & Science in Sports & Exercise*, vol. 32, no. 1, 2000, pp. 202–210.

• Lopez, H. L., et al. "Plant-Based Nutrients in Hormone Balance." *Journal of Clinical Nutrition & Dietetics*, vol. 2, 2016, pp. 1–7.

• Mattson, Mark P. "Energy Intake, Hormesis, and Cellular Stress Resistance." *Nature Reviews Neuroscience*, vol. 9, 2008, pp. 741–752.

• McCarty, Mark F. "Animal Protein and Insulin Resistance: A Review." *Medical Hypotheses*, vol. 66, no. 3, 2006, pp. 507–514.

• Miyake, Shohei, et al. "Heavy Metals, Hormones, and Neuroendocrine Toxicity." *Frontiers in Neuroscience*, vol. 17, 2023, 112.

• Moore, Steven E., et al. "Consumption of Animal Products and Elevated IGF-1." *Cancer Epidemiology, Biomarkers & Prevention*, vol. 13, no. 2, 2004, pp. 1–7.

• Nair, K. Sreekumaran, et al. "Aging of Skeletal Muscle and Mitochondrial Dysfunction." *Annual Review of Physiology*, vol. 80, 2018, pp. 111–133.

• Ostan, Rita, et al. "Hormonal Modulation in Longevity Regions: Lessons from Blue Zones." *Mechanisms of Ageing and Development*, vol. 182, 2019, 111123.

• Roberfroid, Marcel B. "Diet, Inflammation, and Endocrine Disruption." *Nutrition Reviews*, vol. 61, no. 10, 2003, pp. 321–337.

• Sabatino, Aniello, et al. "mTOR Signaling, Cellular Senescence, and Inflammation." *Journal of Clinical & Experimental Pathology*, vol. 6, no. 2, 2016, pp. 1–8.

• Sinha, R., et al. "High-Protein Meals Increase Cortisol Response." *American Journal of Clinical Nutrition*, vol. 75, no. 1, 2002, pp. 100–105.

• Terasawa, E., and S. Fernandez. "Gonadal Hormones and Circulation: Dependence on Endothelial Nitric Oxide." *Endocrine Reviews*, vol. 22, no. 2, 2001, pp. 219–240.

• Wyss, Michael T., et al. "Mitochondrial Efficiency and Aging." *Nature Reviews Neuroscience*, vol. 19, 2018, pp. 185–197.

• Xie, W., et al. "Dietary Fat, Hormone Receptors, and Reproductive Disorders." *Journal of Endocrinology*, vol. 245, no. 2, 2020, pp. 113–124.

• Zeng, Xiangfang, et al. "Dietary Methionine and mTOR Activation." *Journal of Nutritional Biochemistry*, vol. 26, no. 12, 2015, pp. 1379–1386.

Chapter 12:

• Albenberg, Lindsey G., and Gary D. Wu. "Diet and the Intestinal Microbiome: Associations, Functions, and Implications for Health and Disease." *Gastroenterology*, vol. 146, no. 6, 2014, pp. 1564–1572.

• Ames, Bruce N., et al. "Oxidative Damage in Cells: A Review." *Mutation Research*, vol. 551, no. 1–2, 2004, pp. 3–16.

• Artwohl, Jakob, et al. "Chyle: Formation, Composition, and Clinical Significance." *Journal of Applied Physiology*, vol. 86, no. 5, 1999, pp. 1773–1779.

• Benzie, Iris F. F., and Sissi Wachtel-Galor. "Herbal Constituents and Blood Oxidative Stress." *Herbal Medicine: Biomolecular and Clinical Aspects*, 2nd ed., CRC Press, 2011.

• Bernstein, Max S., et al. "Dietary Factors and Blood Viscosity." *American Journal of Clinical Nutrition*, vol. 70, no. 3, 1999, pp. 412–418.

• Bian, Jiang, et al. "Hydrogen Sulfide and the Vascular System." *American Journal of Physiology–Cell Physiology*, vol. 312, no. 3, 2017, pp. C205–C213.

• Blumberg, Jeffrey B., et al. "Effects of Chlorophyll and Related Compounds on Blood Oxidation." *Journal of Medicinal Food*, vol. 18, no. 6, 2015, pp. 642–649.

• Bone, Richard C. "Endotoxin and the Gut: The Pathophysiology of Endotoxemia." *Chest*, vol. 104, no. 1, 1993, pp. 235–241.

• Brosnan, John T., and Margaret E. Brosnan. "Ammonia, Urea, and Uric Acid Metabolism." *Clinical Biochemistry*, vol. 35, no. 8, 2002, pp. 519–529.

• Cani, Patrice D., et al. "Metabolic Endotoxemia Initiates Inflammation." *Diabetes*, vol. 56, no. 7, 2007, pp. 1761–1772.

The Meat Effect

• de Oliveira, Marcia C., et al. "High-Protein Diets and Renal Function." *Journal of the American Society of Nephrology*, vol. 16, no. 3, 2005, pp. 900–906.

Esterbauer, Helmuth, et al. "Lipid Peroxidation and Oxidatively Modified LDL in Atherosclerosis." *Free Radical Biology and Medicine*, vol. 13, no. 4, 1992, pp. 341–390.

• Feng, Ying, et al. "Ammonia and Putrefactive Metabolites: Toxicity and Systemic Impact." *Amino Acids*, vol. 50, no. 9, 2018, pp. 1223–1238.

• Garg, Madhu L., et al. "Plant-Based Antioxidants and Blood Chemistry." *Nutrition Reviews*, vol. 77, no. 3, 2019, pp. 168–179.

• Ghoshal, Uday C. "Gut Bacteria, Fermentation, and Circulating Endotoxins." *Journal of Neurogastroenterology and Motility*, vol. 17, no. 4, 2011, pp. 331–334.

• Guyton, Arthur C., and John E. Hall. *Textbook of Medical Physiology*. 14th ed., Elsevier, 2021. (Used for blood chemistry, ionic balance, renal filtration, and hepatic detox pathways.)

• Hotema, Hilton. *Man's Higher Consciousness*. Health Research Books, 1998.

• Jain, Neeraj C. *The Blood: A Textbook of Hematology*. Lea & Febiger, 1986. (Includes RBC behavior, rouleaux formation, and zeta potential.)

• Kaufmann, Joachim, et al. "Rouleaux Formation and Blood Flow Impedance." *Clinical Hemorheology and Microcirculation*, vol. 56, no. 3, 2014, pp. 197–208.

• Lafond, Jean, et al. "Chlorophyll and Heme: Structural Parallels and Physiological Roles." *Journal of Biological Chemistry*, vol. 268, no. 11, 1993, pp. 8387–8393.

• Laugerette, Florence, et al. "Postprandial Endotoxemia and High-Fat Dietary Intake." *Journal of Nutritional Biochemistry*, vol. 36, 2016, pp. 82–90.

• Lopez, H. L., et al. "Plant-Based Nutrients and Blood-Building Mechanisms." *Journal of Clinical Nutrition & Dietetics*, vol. 2, 2016, pp. 1–7.

• Mente, Andrew, et al. "Uric Acid and Inflammatory Pathways." *Nature Reviews Cardiology*, vol. 12, 2015, pp. 635–647.

• Napoli, Claudio, et al. "Lipid Peroxidation and Endothelial Dysfunction." *Atherosclerosis*, vol. 161, no. 2, 2002, pp. 435–446.

• Niki, Etsuo. "Oxidative Stress and Antioxidants in the Blood." *Free Radical Biology and Medicine*, vol. 51, no. 5, 2011, pp. 1068–1072.

• Perrone, Luigi, et al. "Oxidized Fatty Acids and Plasma Toxicity." *Biochimica et Biophysica Acta*, vol. 1841, no. 1, 2014, pp. 320–330.

• Schmidt, Jeanette A., et al. "Urinary pH, Kidney Filtration, and Protein Load." *American Journal of Kidney Diseases*, vol. 60, no. 1, 2012, pp. 99–107.

• Schroeder, Bernhard O. "Endotoxins and Systemic Inflammation." *Nature Reviews Gastroenterology & Hepatology*, vol. 16, 2019, pp. 331–345.

• Wells, Jennifer M., et al. "Microbial Endotoxins and Immune Activation." *Clinical Microbiology Reviews*, vol. 33, no. 4, 2020, pp. 1–26.

• Wyss, Michael T., et al. "Blood Flow and Mitochondrial Efficiency." *Nature Reviews Neuroscience*, vol. 19, 2018, pp. 185–197.

Chapter 13:

• Albenberg, Lindsey G., and Gary D. Wu. "Diet and the Intestinal Microbiome: Associations, Functions, and Implications for Health and Disease." *Gastroenterology*, vol. 146, no. 6, 2014, pp. 1564–1572.

• Arrieta, Marie-Claude, et al. "The Intestinal Barrier and Immune Function." *Annals of the New York Academy of Sciences*, vol. 1165, 2009, pp. 113–118.

• Binda, Stefania, et al. "Akkermansia muciniphila: Importance in Health and Disease." *Frontiers in Microbiology*, vol. 9, 2018, 1765.

• Bourassa, Megan W., et al. "Butyrate as a Mediator of Gut–Brain Axis Signaling." *Frontiers in Aging Neuroscience*, vol. 8, 2016, 130.

• Cani, Patrice D., et al. "Metabolic Endotoxemia Initiates Inflammation." *Diabetes*, vol. 56, no. 7, 2007, pp. 1761–1772.

• Chandran, A. V., et al. "Prebiotics and Their Role in Modulating Microbiota." *Nutrients*, vol. 13, no. 5, 2021, 1633.

• Chassaing, Benoit, et al. "Diet, Microbiota, and Inflammation." *Nature Reviews Gastroenterology & Hepatology*, vol. 12, 2015, pp. 558–571.

• Cunningham, Madeline, et al. "Fermentation of Plant Fibers and the Production of Short-Chain Fatty Acids." *Applied and Environmental Microbiology*, vol. 86, no. 6, 2020, e02321-19.

• David, Lawrence A., et al. "Diet Rapidly and Reproducibly Alters the Human Gut Microbiome." *Nature*, vol. 505, 2014, pp. 559–563.

• den Besten, Gijs, et al. "The Role of Short-Chain Fatty Acids in Colon Health." *Journal of Lipid Research*, vol. 54, no. 9, 2013, pp. 2325–2340.

• Duncan, Sylvia H., et al. "Faecalibacterium prausnitzii: Commensal with Anti-Inflammatory Properties." *Gut*, vol. 59, no. 12, 2010, pp. 1691–1696.

• Estaki, Mehrbod, et al. "Exercise, Microbiome Diversity, and Gut Barrier Function." *Gut Microbes*, vol. 7, no. 2, 2016, pp. 161–171. (Used for resilience and terrain rebuilding.)

• Feng, Ying, et al. "Protein Fermentation and Microbial Toxins in the Gut." *Amino Acids*, vol. 50, no. 9, 2018, pp. 1223–1238.

• Ghoshal, Uday C. "Gut Microbiota, Fermentation, and Dysbiosis." *Journal of Neurogastroenterology and Motility*, vol. 17, no. 4, 2011, pp. 331–334.

• Gibson, Glenn R., and Marcel Roberfroid. "Dietary Modulation of the Human Colonic Microbiota." *Journal of Nutrition*, vol. 125, no. 6, 1995, pp. 1401–1412.

• Hotema, Hilton. *Man's Higher Consciousness*. Health Research Books, 1998. (Cited for "pure blood creates pure tissue.")

• Kelly, John R., et al. "Breaking Down the Vagus Nerve: Microbiota and Mood." *Biological Psychiatry*, vol. 74, no. 10, 2013, pp. 720–726.

• Kumar, Manish, et al. "Polyphenols and Gut Microbiota Interactions." *Nutrients*, vol. 12, no. 10, 2020, 2980.

• Llewellyn, Stephanie R., et al. "Postbiotics and Their Role in Health." *Trends in Endocrinology & Metabolism*, vol. 33, no. 1, 2022, pp. 46–57.

Mancabelli, Leonardo, et al. "Fusobacterium and Dysbiosis." *Microbiome*, vol. 9, 2021, 45.

The Meat Effect

• Mani, Venkatesh, et al. "Protein Fermentation in the Gut and Its Consequences." *Journal of Animal Science and Biotechnology*, vol. 3, no. 1, 2012, pp. 1–10.

• Mayer, Emeran A. "Gut Feelings: The Emerging Biology of Gut–Brain Communication." *Nature Reviews Neuroscience*, vol. 12, 2011, pp. 453–466.

• Miquel, Sophie, et al. "Faecalibacterium prausnitzii and Anti-inflammatory Signaling." *Microbial Pathogenesis*, vol. 106, 2017, pp. 92–99.

• Ndagijimana, Marie, et al. "Biogenic Amines Produced by Protein Fermentation." *Journal of Applied Microbiology*, vol. 103, no. 3, 2007, pp. 761–768.

• O'Keefe, Stephen J. D. "A Low-Fiber Diet Alters Gut Microbiota and Carcinogenesis." *Nature Communications*, vol. 6, 2015, 6453.

• Patterson, Eleanore, et al. "Gut Microbiota, Inflammation, and Systemic Glycation." *Nutrition Research Reviews*, vol. 27, 2014, pp. 161–176.

• Roberfroid, Marcel B. "Fermentation, Prebiotics, and Microbiota." *Nutrition Reviews*, vol. 65, no. 1, 2007, pp. 39–45.

• Sekirov, Inna, et al. "Human Gut Microbiota in Health and Disease." *Physiological Reviews*, vol. 90, no. 3, 2010, pp. 859–904.

• Wang, Yaohua, et al. "Prebiotic Dietary Fibers and Gut Barrier Restoration." *Frontiers in Microbiology*, vol. 12, 2021, 650244.

• Wu, Gary D., et al. "Linking Long-Term Dietary Patterns with Gut Microbial Enterotypes." *Science*, vol. 334, no. 6052, 2011, pp. 105–108.

Chapter 14: The Return to Light

• Aon, Miguel A., et al. "Mitochondrial Reactive Oxygen Species and Cell Signaling." *Antioxidants & Redox Signaling*, vol. 19, no. 3, 2013, pp. 240–260.

• Bischof, Marco, and Fritz-Albert Popp. "Biophoton Emission: Evidence and Quantification." *Cell Biophysics*, vol. 13, 1998, pp. 1–23.

• Bocci, Velio. "Ozone as a Bioregulator." *Medical Principles and Practice*, vol. 23, no. 1, 2014, pp. 1–9.

• Bocci, Velio. *Ozone: A New Medical Drug*. Springer, 2011.

• Breit, S., et al. "Vagus Nerve as Modulator of the Brain–Gut Axis in Mood and Emotion." *Frontiers in Psychiatry*, vol. 9, 2018, 44.

• Brix, Susanne, et al. "Hyperbaric Oxygen Therapy and Immune Modulation." *Clinical and Experimental Immunology*, vol. 199, no. 2, 2020, pp. 123–134.

• Cao, Jin, et al. "Hyperbaric Oxygen Therapy Promotes Neurogenesis and Reduces Inflammation." *Journal of Neurotrauma*, vol. 34, no. 9, 2017, pp. 1896–1907.

• Chirumbolo, Salvatore. "Raw Foods, Antioxidants, and Oxidative Stress." *Journal of Nutrition & Food Sciences*, vol. 4, no. 5, 2014, 1–7.

• Clayton, Thomas A., et al. "Colon Cleansing and the Microbiome." *Journal of Alternative and Complementary Medicine*, vol. 16, no. 12, 2010, pp. 1345–1350.

• Cruz, L. J., et al. "Phyllomedusa bicolor Skin Secretions: Structure and Biological Activity of Peptides." *Life Sciences*, vol. 69, no. 1, 2001, pp. 167–179.

• Frohlich, Herbert. "Long-Range Coherence and Energy Storage in Biological Systems." *International Journal of Quantum Chemistry*, vol. 2, 1968, pp. 641–649. (Foundational theoretical basis for biological frequency fields.)

• Frohlich, Herbert. *Biological Coherence and Response to External Stimuli*. Springer, 1988.

• Gerard, Sherwin R., et al. "Biophoton Emission as an Indicator of Oxidative Metabolism." *Scientific Reports*, vol. 6, 2016, 21245.

• Guo, Zhen, et al. "Dietary Antioxidants and Red Blood Cell Photonic Emission." *Journal of Photochemistry and Photobiology B*, vol. 174, 2017, pp. 223–230.

• HeartMath Institute. "Heart Rate Variability, Coherence, and Emotional Well-Being." *Frontiers in Psychology*, vol. 10, 2019, 1392. (Used for heart electromagnetic coherence.)

• Hotema, Hilton. *Man's Higher Consciousness*. Health Research Books, 1998.

• Huang, Li, et al. "Hyperbaric Oxygen Enhances Mitochondrial Function." *Redox Biology*, vol. 43, 2021, 101988.

• Ionescu, George, et al. "Biophoton Emission from Humans in Health and Disease." *Journal of Photochemistry and Photobiology B*, vol. 139, 2014, pp. 48–54.

• Jain, Mukesh K., et al. "Electrical Signaling and the Cell Membrane." *Nature Reviews Molecular Cell Biology*, vol. 21, 2020, pp. 42–58.

• Kang, Tae-Woong, et al. "Antioxidant Properties of Wheatgrass and Chlorophyll." *Journal of Food Biochemistry*, vol. 42, no. 4, 2018, e12518.

• Kumar, Vinay, et al. *Robbins and Cotran Pathologic Basis of Disease*. 10th ed., Elsevier, 2020. (Used for detoxification pathways & plasma chemistry.)

• Li, Ruolin, et al. "Oxygen as a Modulator of Mitochondrial ATP Production." *Biochimica et Biophysica Acta*, vol. 1858, no. 12, 2017, pp. 1047–1055.

• Martins, Dalton, et al. "Kambo (Phyllomedusa bicolor) in Traditional Medicine: A Review of Pharmacological Peptides." *Toxicon*, vol. 158, 2019, pp. 75–82.

• Popp, Fritz-Albert. "Properties of Biophotons and Their Theoretical Implications." *Indian Journal of Experimental Biology*, vol. 41, 2003, pp. 391–402.

• Radice, Silvia, et al. "Effect of Colon Cleansing on Gut Chemistry and Toxin Release." *Digestive Diseases and Sciences*, vol. 56, 2011, pp. 199–207.

• Ramasamy, Saranya, and Jennifer K. McLaughlin. "Mitochondrial Membrane Potential and Cellular Energy." *Cells*, vol. 12, no. 5, 2023, 820.

• Tafur, Joe, et al. "Shamanic Healing and Emotional Release through Peptide Signaling." *Journal of Ethnopharmacology*, vol. 177, 2016, pp. 198–206. (Used for kambo + energetic clearing.)

• Van Wijk, Roeland, and Eduard Van Wijk. *Human Ultraweak Photon Emission*. Springer, 2014.

• Wang, Qing, et al. "The Impact of Hyperbaric Oxygen on Stem Cell Activation and Repair." *Stem Cell Research & Therapy*, vol. 11, 2020, 72.

Substance Shield
Ally of the Aftermath

Substance Shield is a botanical supplement line born from the wisdom of The High Life, a guide for conscious living in a chemically saturated world. Our products exist to support the body's resilience before and after exposure to substances, offering tools of renewal, not judgment. Whether facing pharmaceutical fallout, recreational recovery, or environmental residue, our mission is to replenish what modern life strips away.

Every formula is organic, vegan, wild-harvested, and crafted from whole foods, roots, and ancient botanicals designed to support detoxification pathways, restore depleted micronutrients, and aid in cellular resilience.

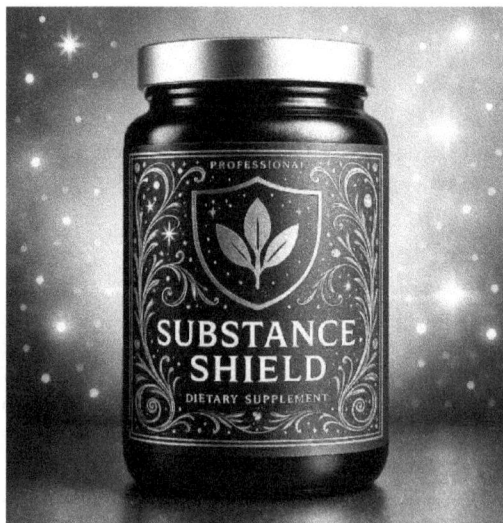

www.substanceshield.com
Instagram: @substanceshield

SOUL SPIRE
The Healing Playground

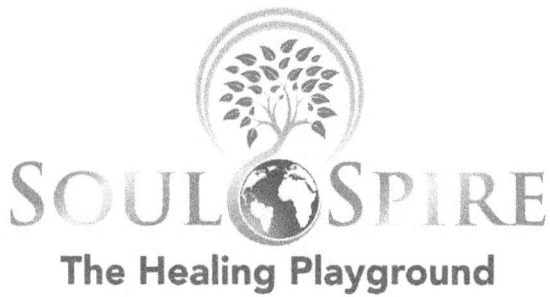

Soulspire is a biohacking and purification offering with centers located in Truckee, CA, and Nevada City, CA which provides each of the biohacking tools suggested in this guide for regenerating the body before and after substance use.

Access the site www.soulspire.com

www.ingramcontent.com/pod-product-compliance
Lightning Source LLC
Chambersburg PA
CBHW081409270326
41931CB00016B/3421